Small Incision Lenticule Extraction (SMILE)

Surgical Technique and Challenges

Comprehensive Text and Video Guide

System requirement:

Windows:

- Operating System:
  - Windows Vista or above
  - Macintosh OS X or above
- Recommended Web Browser – Google Chrome & Mozilla Firefox
- Essential plugins – Java & Flash player
  - If facing problems in viewing content – enable/re-install Java plugin on your web browser setting.
  - If Videos don't show up – enable/re-install Flash Player or manage Flash setting on your web browser settings.
  - You can test Java and Flash by using the links from the help section of the CD/DVD.

Accompanying CD/DVD Rom is compatible and playable only in Computers and not in DVD player.

CD/DVD has Autorun function (*only for Windows based systems*). If Autorun feature doesn't work, then follow the steps below to access the contents manually:

Windows:

- Click on My Computer
- Select the CD/DVD drive and click open/explore – this will show list of files in the CD/DVD
- Find and double click file – "launch.html"

Mac:

Double click the file "launch.html" located on the root after inserting the CD/DVD. The Mac OSX operating system does not support an Autorun feature.

For more information about troubleshoot of Autorun click on:
http://support.microsoft.com/kb/330135

Small Incision Lenticule Extraction (SMILE)

Surgical Technique and Challenges

Comprehensive Text and Video Guide

Editors

Jeewan S Titiyal MD
Professor and Head
Cornea, Cataract and Refractive Surgery Services
Dr Rajendra Prasad Centre for Ophthalmic Sciences
All India Institute of Medical Sciences
New Delhi, India

Manpreet Kaur MD
Research Associate
Cornea, Cataract and Refractive Surgery Services
Dr Rajendra Prasad Centre for Ophthalmic Sciences
All India Institute of Medical Sciences
New Delhi, India

Foreword

Walter Sekundo

JAYPEE The Health Sciences Publisher
New Delhi | London | Panama

Jaypee Brothers Medical Publishers (P) Ltd

Headquarters
Jaypee Brothers Medical Publishers (P) Ltd.
4838/24, Ansari Road, Daryaganj
New Delhi 110 002, India
Phone: +91-11-43574357
Fax: +91-11-43574314
E-mail: jaypee@jaypeebrothers.com

Overseas Offices

J.P. Medical Ltd.
83, Victoria Street, London
SW1H 0HW (UK)
Phone: +44-20 3170 8910
Fax: +44(0)20 3008 6180
E-mail: info@jpmedpub.com

Jaypee-Highlights Medical Publishers Inc.
City of Knowledge, Bld. 235, 2nd Floor, Clayton
Panama City, Panama
Phone: +1 507-301-0496
Fax: +1 507-301-0499
E-mail: cservice@jphmedical.com

Jaypee Brothers Medical Publishers (P) Ltd.
17/1-B, Babar Road, Block-B, Shaymali
Mohammadpur, Dhaka-1207
Bangladesh
Mobile: +08801912003485
E-mail: jaypeedhaka@gmail.com

Jaypee Brothers Medical Publishers (P) Ltd.
Bhotahity, Kathmandu, Nepal
Phone: +977-9741283608
E-mail: kathmandu@jaypeebrothers.com

Website: www.jaypeebrothers.com
Website: www.jaypeedigital.com

Small Incision Lenticule Extraction (SMILE)
Surgical Technique and Challenges
Comprehensive Text and Video Guide

First Edition: **2018**

ISBN: 978-93-5270-214-5

Printed at Ajanta Offset & Packagings Ltd., Faridabad, Haryana

Dedicated to

My parents, My dear wife Basanti Titiyal
My children, Dr Hemant Titiyal and Dr Renuka Titiyal

Jeewan S Titiyal

My Alma Mater and my mentors, for being the guiding light
My family, for their unwavering support, love and time

Manpreet Kaur

Our patients, who constantly inspire us to perform better

Jeewan S Titiyal & Manpreet Kaur

Contributors

Anand Singh Brar MBBS
Junior Resident
Dr Rajendra Prasad Centre for
Ophthalmic Sciences
All India Institute of Medical Sciences
New Delhi, India

Ruchita Falera MD
Senior Resident
Cornea, Cataract and Refractive
Surgery Services
Dr Rajendra Prasad Centre for
Ophthalmic Sciences
All India Institute of Medical Sciences
New Delhi, India

Manpreet Kaur MD
Research Associate
Cornea, Cataract and Refractive
Surgery Services
Dr Rajendra Prasad Centre for
Ophthalmic Sciences
All India Institute of Medical Sciences
New Delhi, India

Krishna Prasad Kudlu MS
Medical Director
Prasad Netralaya
Udupi, Mangalore, Sullia, Thirtahalli
Karnataka, India

Sridevi Nair MD
Senior Resident
Cornea, Cataract and Refractive
Surgery Services
Dr Rajendra Prasad Centre for
Ophthalmic Sciences
All India Institute of Medical Sciences
New Delhi, India

Anubha Rathi MD
Senior Resident
Cornea, Cataract and Refractive
Surgery Services
Dr Rajendra Prasad Centre for
Ophthalmic Sciences
All India Institute of Medical Sciences
New Delhi, India

Mahipal S Sachdev MD
Chairman and Medical Director
Centre for Sight Group of Eye Hospitals
New Delhi, India

Ritika Sachdev MS
Additional Director of Medical Services
Centre for Sight Group of Eye Hospitals
New Delhi, India

Ramkishor Sah PhD (Ophthalmology)
Scholar
Scientist-I
Contact Lens Services
Dr Rajendra Prasad Centre for
Ophthalmic Sciences
All India Institute of Medical Sciences
New Delhi, India

Pranita Sahay MD
Senior Resident
Cornea, Cataract and Refractive
Surgery Services
Dr Rajendra Prasad Centre for
Ophthalmic Sciences
All India Institute of Medical Sciences
New Delhi, India

Harathy Selvan MBBS
Junior Resident
Dr Rajendra Prasad Centre for
Ophthalmic Sciences
All India Institute of Medical Sciences
New Delhi, India

Rupal Shah MS
Group Medical Director
Centre for Sight-New Vision Laser Centres
Vadodara, Gujarat, India

Jeewan S Titiyal MD
Professor and Head
Cornea, Cataract and Refractive
Surgery Services
Dr Rajendra Prasad Centre for
Ophthalmic Sciences
All India Institute of Medical Sciences
New Delhi, India

Foreword

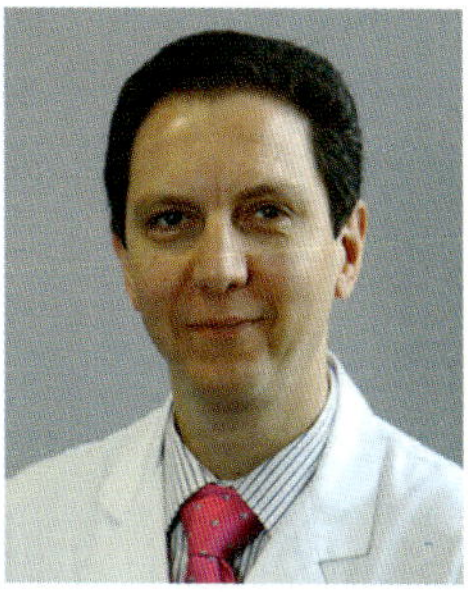

Roughly a decade ago, a new 'kid on the block' appeared in the field of corneal refractive surgery. For the first time, it seemed possible that another type of laser, the femtosecond laser, could challenge the overall predominance of excimer laser technology. The development of this new procedure, which was named Small Incision Lenticule Extraction (SMILE), is also closely related to Indian ophthalmology, since the primary steps of this procedure were undertaken in India right after the initial trials in Germany.

While being criticized in the early stages, this new procedure has swiftly gained popularity in the last years, and since the recent FDA approval in 2016 became truly embraced by the world of ophthalmology. Meanwhile, almost one million registered SMILE procedures have been performed worldwide, and new SMILE surgeons enter the market virtually month by month. However, unlike Femto-Lasik, the surgical procedure of SMILE is technically more difficult, requires better manual surgical skills, and may be especially challenging for the beginner.

So far, only one book on SMILE has been published in English, whereas one was released in Chinese, and the third is due to appear in Spanish.

So why another book on SMILE, and what makes this book so unique and worth reading it? Unlike other books written by a large cohort of contributors from all over the world, this present work has been done by a small group of dedicated refractive surgeons with their personal view, enriched by a thorough study of the literature. This makes this publication a real 'one to one guide' for the beginners and more advanced SMILE surgeons alike.

Indeed, the authors provide a step-by-step written and video-assisted guidance of the surgical technique, highlighting the crucial steps. Moreover, the various complications that come along with new technology and may be encountered during the surgery or thereafter, are not only explained in detail, but the management and prevention are clearly and precisely explained. The most prominent feature is not only a good and understandable language of the chapters but nicely prepared, concise tables and self-explanatory diagrams. The clinical pictures and the images of high quality also help to gain the necessary knowledge swiftly and effectively.

The book is divided into 12 chapters, starting with a nice introduction to the history of lasers in refractive surgery, leading to the development of

Femtosecond lasers. Subsequently, the authors provide a practical guide for patient selection with an overview of the decision process, as to who is a good candidate for SMILE surgery and who should be offered other means of laser correction. I also recommend a chapter where the principles of the laser machine and the parameters are explained, because a good corneal refractive surgeon who wants to achieve great outcomes with SMILE cannot rely on the company instructors alone. The surgeon needs to understand every change that is nowadays possible using Expert Mode in order to assure a smooth laser dissection depending upon age, gender and the degree of ametropia.

Thereafter, the expected outcomes, visual recovery and other features you want to know when counseling your patients are explained in depths. The chapters on complications and laser energy management are both well written and illustrative, using tables for quick reference. Last but not least, enhancement strategies and an up-to-date review of lenticule use beyond standard SMILE are described.

The highlight of this book, however, is the impressive collection of surgical videos with integrated animations.

In summary, this book written by a dedicated group of clinicians from New Delhi will serve as a quick reference point and a comprehensive guide for the novice and more experienced SMILE surgeons, helping them in their daily work, reducing complications, and enhancing the comprehension of this great procedure. I am very grateful to Dr Titiyal, Dr Kaur, and their colleagues from All India Institute of Medical Sciences, New Delhi, for their gift to the refractive community, and can highly recommend this book to my colleagues.

This book will be useful to all of us!

Walter Sekundo MD PhD
Professor of Ophthalmology
Marburg, Germany

Preface

The field of refractive surgery has witnessed a paradigm shift with the introduction of femtosecond laser technology in 2001. Over the last few years, the flap-based corneal ablative procedures have given way to flapless refractive lenticule extraction.

Small Incision Lenticule Extraction (SMILE) has recently received FDA approval in 2016, and is increasingly becoming the procedure of choice for the correction of myopia and myopic astigmatism. The world is currently in the transition phase, with surgeons shifting from *Laser-Assisted In Situ Keratomileusis (LASIK)* to *Small Incision Lenticule Extraction (SMILE)*. An in-depth understanding of the procedure, its outcomes, as well as the intra-operative challenges is essential before embarking on this new procedure.

At present, there is a paucity of literature providing a comprehensive overview of the surgery with its associated complications. The book will serve as a quick reference point for refractive surgeons performing SMILE, and provide surgical pearls to enhance understanding. The highlight of this book is its impressive video collection, encompassing the surgical techniques of surgeons well-versed with the procedure, intraoperative difficulties faced during the initial learning curve and their management. We have provided a step-by-step video-assisted guidance to master the surgical steps with ease. Surgical techniques of some of the experienced surgeons have been incorporated in this book in order to broaden the perspective. Animations have been integrated with the videos to facilitate clarity of concepts.

SMILE has a steep learning curve, and we have provided a comprehensive review of the complications, as well as their management to ease the flap to cap transition. The text is interspersed with easy to understand, concise tables, self-explanatory diagrams, clinical pictures and anterior segment optical coherence tomography (ASOCT) images to recapitulate the salient points and enhance understanding.

We have also discussed the exciting future prospects of this novel procedure, as well as the potential applications of the refractive lenticule thus extracted.

The book should be extremely useful to the refractive surgeons, as well as the training institutions. We hope, our readers and viewers will be able to apply the surgical tips to simplify the learning process of an initially challenging procedure and smile their way to success. The book will be an invaluable asset for all refractive surgeons and serve as a one-point reference to provide day-to-day guidance.

Jeewan S Titiyal
Manpreet Kaur

Acknowledgments

We express our sincere gratitude to the entire staff of our Cornea and Refractive Investigative Laboratory, who were of invaluable help in the meticulous maintenance of the clinical records.

Our heartfelt thanks to the entire CMET team involved in the recording of the surgical videos. We wish to thank the staff of the SMILE operation theater for providing an organized and efficient working environment.

We thank all our colleagues and residents of the Cornea and Refractive Surgery Units for their support. We also wish to thank all our contributors for their valuable efforts.

We wish to acknowledge the commendable efforts of the Zeiss technical team and application specialists at every step of this venture.

We sincerely appreciate the entire production team of Jaypee Brothers Medical Publishers for their exemplary hard-work, support and commitment towards this project.

Contents

1. **Evolution of Femtosecond Laser Technology in Refractive Surgery** 1
   Sridevi Nair, Manpreet Kaur, Jeewan S Titiyal
2. **Patient Counseling and Preoperative Evaluation** 9
   Sridevi Nair, Manpreet Kaur, Jeewan S Titiyal
3. **Corneal Wound Healing, Morphological and Biomechanical Changes after Small Incision Lenticule Extraction** 21
   Pranita Sahay, Manpreet Kaur, Anand Singh Brar, Jeewan S Titiyal
4. **Understanding the Machine and Laser Settings** 32
   Anubha Rathi, Manpreet Kaur, Jeewan S Titiyal
5. **Surgical Technique of Small Incision Lenticule Extraction** 46
   Manpreet Kaur, Jeewan S Titiyal
6. **Stepwise Approach for Beginners: Navigating the Learning Curve** 65
   Anubha Rathi, Manpreet Kaur, Jeewan S Titiyal
7. **Refractive and Physiological Outcomes of Small Incision Lenticule Extraction** 77
   Pranita Sahay, Manpreet Kaur, Jeewan S Titiyal
8. **Intraoperative Complications in Small Incision Lenticule Extraction** 88
   Manpreet Kaur, Jeewan S Titiyal
9. **Postoperative Complications in Small Incision Lenticule Extraction** 113
   Ruchita Falera, Manpreet Kaur, Anand Singh Brar, Jeewan S Titiyal
10. **Post-SMILE Enhancement and Retreatment** 137
    Manpreet Kaur, Jeewan S Titiyal
11. **SMILE versus Femtosecond LASIK: Weighing the Pros and Cons** 148
    Anubha Rathi, Manpreet Kaur, Anand Singh Brar, Ramkishor Sah, Jeewan S Titiyal
12. **Future Technological Advances in Small Incision Lenticule Extraction** 161
    Harathy Selvan, Manpreet Kaur, Jeewan S Titiyal

Index *175*

DVD Contents

SURGICAL TECHNIQUE

Jeewan S Titiyal

Video 1: Surgical Technique of Small Incision Lenticule Extraction (3 mm side-cut)

- Docking
- Infrared centration check
- Femtosecond laser application
- Opening the side-cut and lenticule edge identification
- Lenticule dissection
- Lenticule extraction
- Examining the lenticule
- Ensuring cap apposition
- Slit illumination to examine interface

Video 2: Docking: Technique, Challenges and Complications

- Selection of treatment pack and its attachment
- Ideal docking
- Interface and its importance
- Centration check and challenges
- Difficult docking and suction loss

Video 3: Opening the Cap Side-cut

- Gentle massage to highlight the edges
- Superficial opening of the incision
- Epithelial defect due to inadvertent sub-epithelial entry

Video 4: Identifying the Lenticule Edge

- Identifying the lenticule edge in 2 mm incisions
- Identifying the lenticule edge in 3 mm incisions
- Identifying the lenticule edge in 4 mm incisions

Video 5: Lenticule Dissection

- Identifying the correct planes and smooth lenticule dissection
- Lenticule dissection with shaft like lamellar dissector
- Shifting from shaft like dissector to spoon shaped dissector
- Lenticule folded in half with difficult dissection
- Microadhesions with difficult dissection
- Difficulty identifying the second dissection plane
- Cap-lenticular adhesions

Video 6: Lenticule Extraction
- Forceps assisted lenticule extraction
- Difficulty in grasping the lenticule
- Enhancing edge to facilitate grasping
- Dissector assisted lenticule extraction
- Difficult lenticule extraction
- Two side-cuts to extract lenticule
- Cap tear during lenticule extraction
- Lenticule extraction with retained fragments

Video 7: After Lenticule Extraction
- Examine the lenticule
- Irrigate interface
- Smoothen the cap
- Slit-illumination

Video 8: Surgical Technique of Small Incision Lenticule Extraction (2 mm side-cut)

Video 9: Surgical Technique of Small Incision Lenticule Extraction (4 mm side-cut)

Video 10: Surgical Technique of Small Incision Lenticule Extraction (Two side-cuts)

INTRAOPERATIVE COMPLICATIONS

Jeewan S Titiyal

Video 11: Suction Loss
- Suction loss immediately after docking
- Suction loss during lenticule cut

Video 12: Black Spots
- Interface debris with black spots
- Air in interface with black spots

Video 13: Opaque Bubble Layer
- OBL with difficult dissection
- OBL extending up to limbus
- OBL in a case with entrapped conjunctiva in suction ring
- OBL in 2 mm incision

Video 14: Lenticule Mis-dissection and Cap-Lenticular Adhesions
- Cap-lenticular adhesion with retained lenticule
- Sinskey method to manage cap-lenticular adhesions

Video 15: Partially Retained Lenticule Fragments

Video 16: Cap and Side-cut Tears

- Cap tear
- Side-cut extension
- Side-cut tear

Video 17: Epithelial Defect

RETREATMENT

Video 18: Thin-flap LASIK after SMILE

Jeewan S Titiyal

Video 19: Circle Pattern of VisuMax Laser

Mahipal S Sachdev, Ritika Sachdev

MISCELLANEOUS

Video 20: Small Incision Lenticule Extraction (SMILE): Surgical Technique and Challenging Situations

Rupal Shah

Video 21: Step-wise Approach for Beginners: FLEx and Pseudo-SMILE

Krishna Prasad Kudlu

Chapter 1

Evolution of Femtosecond Laser Technology in Refractive Surgery

Sridevi Nair, Manpreet Kaur, Jeewan S Titiyal

INTRODUCTION

The history of medicine is replete with instances of path-breaking discoveries and inventions, which have had a significant impact on mankind. *Light amplification by stimulated emission of radiation (LASER)* is an instance of one such landmark development, which has changed the management of numerous diseases in the field of medicine, especially in ophthalmology. We have briefly outlined the evolution of lasers in ophthalmology, with an emphasis on femtosecond laser technology. The changing paradigm of cornea-based refractive surgeries has been described, from the early mechanical reshaping of the cornea to the present day flapless femtosecond laser-assisted refractive lenticule extraction (Flowchart 1.1).

LASERS IN OPHTHALMOLOGY: A BRIEF HISTORY

Today, one tends to associate the term LASER with precision, accuracy and speed. However, its evolution has taken decades of work by numerous scientists around the world. The use of light as a therapeutic agent in ophthalmology dates back to the 1940s, when Meyer-Schwickerath first focused strong sunlight on the retina of patients with choroidal melanomas in order to treat them.[1] The concept of stimulated emission was introduced by Einstein in 1917.[2] Townes and Schawlow used microwave radiation as the external source for stimulated emission and developed *microwave amplification by stimulated emission of radiation (MASER)*. Gordon provided the concept of using light as the source for stimulated emission, and thus coined the term *light amplification by stimulated emission of radiation* or LASER.[3]

Laser radiation has the advantage of being highly coherent, monochromatic and collimated. The first functional laser was developed by Maiman in 1960.[4] Zaret produced the first ocular lesion using ruby laser in 1961.[5] In 1964, Bridges developed the argon laser with emission in the blue and green wavelengths.[6] In 1970, Basov built a laser using xenon dimer gas, and called it excimer laser (an abbreviation for excited dimer).[7] Argon fluoride laser, a type

Flowchart 1.1: Evolution of corneal refractive surgery.

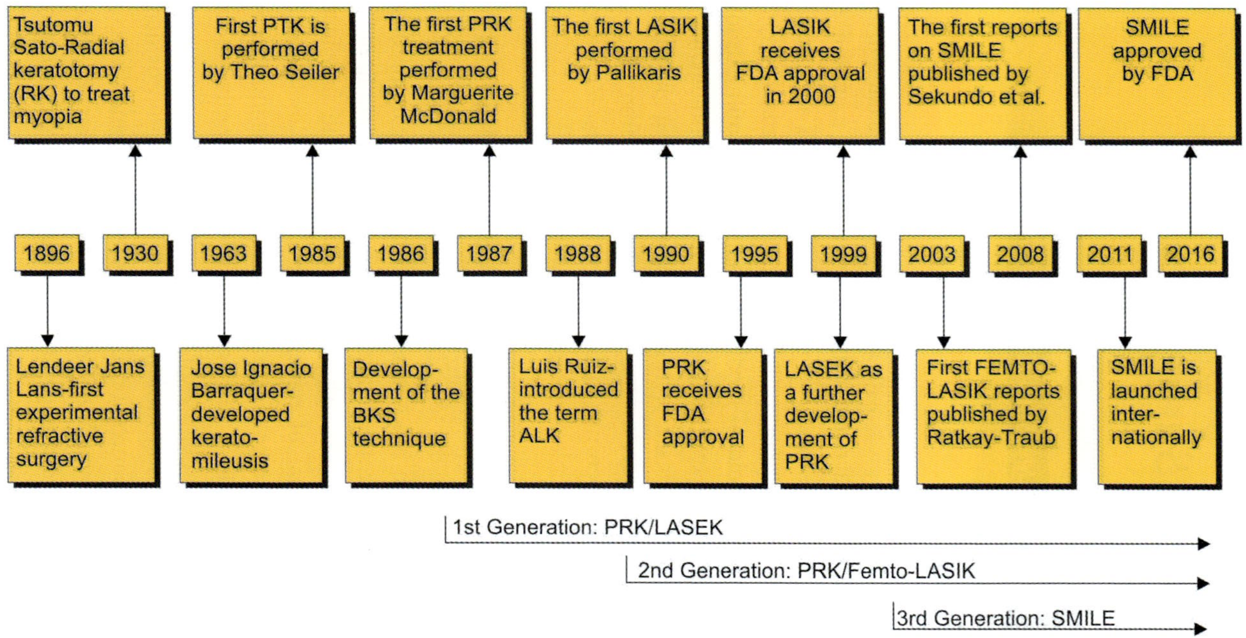

(PTK: Phototherapeutic keratectomy; BKS: Barraquer-Krumeich-Swinger; ALK: Automated lamellar keratoplasty; PRK: Photorefractive keratectomy; FDA: Food and Drug Administration; LASEK: Laser-assisted subepithelial keratomileusis; SMILE: Small incision lenticule extraction; LASIK: Laser-assisted in situ keratomileusis).

of excimer laser, was developed in 1976, with emission in the ultraviolet range at a wavelength of 193 nm.[8]

CORNEAL REFRACTIVE SURGERY: TRACING THE BEGINNING

The history of corneal refractive surgery dates back to the year 1896, when Lendeer Jans Lans gave the idea of reshaping the cornea for correcting corneal astigmatism using penetrating corneal cuts. He concluded that traverse incisions flattened the cornea in the meridian perpendicular to the incisions.[9]

Decades later, in the 1930s, Tsutomu Sato conceptualized this principle in the form of the technique of radial keratotomy, a procedure which was later popularized by Fyodorov et al. Sato had observed a flattening effect in the cornea of keratoconus patients after an episode of acute hydrops. He subsequently created both anterior and posterior corneal incisions to cause flattening in order to correct myopia. Radial keratotomy gained immense popularity during the 1970s and 1980s for the surgical correction of myopia.[10]

In 1964, Jose Ignacio Barraquer, belonging to the third generation of a family of famous ophthalmologists in Spain, introduced the idea of keratomileusis, which literally meant *corneal carving*. He used a manual microkeratome for lamellar dissection of cornea. The disc, thus obtained, was frozen (with liquid nitrogen or solid carbon dioxide) and cryolathed on its posterior surface based on the refractive correction required. This disc was then sutured onto the corneal stromal bed. However, the technique was not very suitable to correct astigmatism.[11] Later on, his pupils developed the Barraquer-Krumeich-Swinger (BKS) nonfreeze technique, which did not require the freezing of the dissected corneal disc, thereby leading to fewer postoperative complications and faster visual recovery.[12] Ruiz modified the technique by doing an in situ keratomileusis, wherein he resected a layer of tissue from the stromal bed itself by passing the microkeratome at a different depth after making the initial cap. He is also credited with the development of an automated microkeratome, producing a more regular corneal surface with greater precision. He demonstrated the formation of a corneal flap by stopping the microkeratome head before the end of the pass, followed by stromal bed resection and repositioning of the flap. This helped in avoiding the cap related complications.[13,14]

The introduction of argon fluoride laser in 1981 heralded a major breakthrough in the field of refractive surgery. It allowed enhanced precision levels and led to the creation of clean, etched-out lesions with minimal collateral damage.

The utility of excimer laser was subsequently expanded to radial keratotomy as well as photorefractive keratectomy (PRK).[15-18]

Pallikaris described the present technique of laser-assisted in situ keratomileusis (LASIK) in 1991. He created a hinged corneal flap using a guarded microkeratome followed by excimer laser-assisted stromal ablation.[19]

The late 1980s and early 1990s witnessed an increasing use of picosecond and nanosecond lasers for in situ keratomileusis and corneal flap creation. These lasers were the precursors of femtosecond lasers, which were introduced in the subsequent decade.

In 1996, Ito et al. attempted the use of a 1,053 nm picosecond laser (10^{-12}) to create a corneal flap as well as a stromal lenticule in experimental rabbit eyes. The infrared picosecond laser replaced the functions of microkeratome and excimer laser, and this experimental technique formed the basis of refractive lenticule extraction by Sekundo et al. in 2008.[20] In 1998, Krueger et al. used the picosecond laser [Neodymium-doped yttrium lithium fluoride (Nd:YLF), 1053 nm; energy: 25 μJ/pulse, 30 picoseconds] in a case with –15 D myopia to create the corneal flap and perform excimer laser-assisted stromal ablation. They also attempted both flap creation and stromal lenticule creation [again, a precursor to femtosecond lenticule extraction (FLEx)] with the picosecond laser.[21] Krueger et al. (1996) evaluated the corneal stroma ultrastructure after picosecond laser photodisruption and observed multiple, coalescing intrastromal cavities parallel to the corneal surface, without any thermal necrosis or coagulative change in the region of tissue interaction.[22] The incision quality and precision produced by picosecond lasers were comparable to that produced by excimer laser.[23]

FEMTOSECOND LASERS IN CORNEAL REFRACTIVE SURGERY

Femtosecond lasers in ophthalmology were introduced by Kurtz et al. in 1998, who created corneal flaps in primate cadaver eyes with high precision and smooth lamellar dissection planes.[24] Dr Tibor Juhasz and his team are credited with designing and building the first surgical ophthalmic femtosecond laser system. He worked in collaboration with Dr Kurtz and his associates to develop the laser parameters for use in corneal refractive surgery.[25] Laser pulses of ultrashort duration of the order of 10^{-15} seconds were focused 150–200 microns below the epithelial surface and delivered in a spiral pattern. Tissue dissection was achieved best at pulse energies ranging from 4 μJ to 8 μJ and spot separations of 10–15 microns.

The first Food and Drug Administration (FDA) approved femtosecond laser for ophthalmological use was IntraLase Pulsion. It was approved in the year 2000 for lamellar corneal surgery and became commercially available for creation of corneal flap in LASIK surgery by 2001. The laser spots were delivered in a spiral pattern. The earlier models were of the low frequency and high energy. The first generation IntraLase Pulsion femtosecond laser

(Abbott Medical Optics) had a frequency of only about 10 kHz. With technological advancements, higher frequencies and lower energies were targeted. This translated to greater cutting speeds, more efficient tissue cutting and less spill-over effect on the adjacent tissue. The second and third generation IntraLase laser systems had a frequency of 15 kHz and 30 kHz, respectively, while the energy delivered lowered to 2.9 μJ and 1.7 μJ. The lower energy systems require closer spacing of the laser spots. The fifth generation IntraLase femtolaser received FDA approval in 2008 for FS-LASIK (Femtosecond-LASIK). It had a planar applanation system with a frequency of 150 kHz and could create a flap in about 10 seconds.

In 2007, VisuMax laser (200 kHz) was approved for its laser microkeratome function by the FDA. The currently available VisuMax laser (Carl Zeiss Meditec AG) has a frequency of 500 kHz with each pulse conveying energy of about 150 nJ. The laser spots have 1 μm diameter and are placed at a distance of 2–5 μm in a spiral pattern. The VisuMax laser, unlike the IntraLase, has a curved applanation surface which causes less corneal distortion and minimizes intraocular pressure (IOP) spikes. The other femtosecond laser systems approved for femto-LASIK include the Femtec (Technolas Perfect Vision), Femto LDV (Ziemer Ophthalmic Systems AG), and Wavelight FS200 (Alcon Surgical).

The femtosecond laser technology has evolved from the early laser systems with a low repetition rate (10 kHz) which needed higher energy to operate, to the newer devices having a higher repetition rate (as high as 500 kHz), with lesser energy utilization, shorter procedure duration and better surface quality.[26] In addition to refractive surgery, femtosecond lasers have found applications in tunnel creation for intracorneal ring segments (INTACS), astigmatic keratotomy, keratoplasty (both penetrating and lamellar) and cataract surgery.

The femtosecond lasers were a major advancement over the microkeratome in being able to make thinner flaps which were more precise and thus, associated with fewer flap-related complications and corneal biomechanical changes.[27]

In the year 2000, Holger et al. used Ti-sapphire femtosecond laser in porcine eyes to create corneal flaps and stromal lenticules. They observed enhanced precision of stromal cuts with pulse energies of 1–2 μJ (lower than that used by Kurtz et al.), spot size of 5–10 microns and spot separation of 8 microns. The thermal alteration of adjacent tissue was of the order of only 1 micron.[28] Subsequently, in 2003, Heisterkamp et al. successfully demonstrated the use of femtosecond laser in rabbit corneas for creation of the anterior corneal flap and stromal lenticule, which was extracted after lifting the flap. They proposed femtosecond laser to be a suitable replacement for both microkeratome and excimer laser.[29]

In 2003, Ratkay-Traub et al. published the clinical results of use of femtosecond neodymium-glass laser on human eyes. It was used to create the corneal flap, perform keratomileusis and create channels for intrastromal ring segments. Comparable results were observed between FS-LASIK and microkeratome-LASIK. Femtosecond laser created precise stromal cuts with additional advantages over the mechanical methods.[30]

The evolution of refractive lenticule extraction marked the next major breakthrough in the field of refractive surgery. Sekundo et al. introduced the technique of FLEx in 2008, which involved a femtosecond laser-assisted creation of a flap as well as a refractive lenticule. The femtosecond laser flap was lifted akin to the LASIK flap, and the underlying refractive lenticule was dissected from the stromal bed and extracted.[31] At present, the VisuMax (Carl Zeiss Meditec, Jena, Germany) laser platform is the only commercially available system that allows refractive lenticule creation. Though the new procedure of refractive lenticule extraction was observed to be safe and efficacious, it did not lead to a decrease in the flap-related complications.[32] There was a need for superior procedures that eliminated the need for a corneal flap. This led to the evolution of small incision lenticule extraction (SMILE) in 2010. Sekundo et al. described the creation of an intrastromal refractive lenticule that could be extracted through two small side-cut incisions of 80° chord length, placed 180° apart. Although the lenticule dissection and extraction is more challenging, the technique is associated with a significantly decreased incidence of microstriae and dry eyes as well as an improved internal structural stability. SMILE became available for commercial use in 2011.[33]

The initial VisuMax laser system used for SMILE had a frequency of 200 kHz. The new 500 kHz VisuMax femtosecond laser received the FDA approval for SMILE in September 2016. It is currently approved to treat myopia ranging from –1.00 D to -8.00 D of myopia, with less than or equal to –0.50 D cylinder and manifest refraction spherical equivalent (MRSE) less than or equal to –8.25 D. It is not yet approved for treating astigmatism or hyperopia. Currently, trials are ongoing to evaluate the safety and efficacy of SMILE in higher degrees of myopia, as well as astigmatism and hyperopia.

CONCLUSION

Femtosecond laser technology was introduced in the field of refractive surgery in 2001 for the creation of lamellar corneal flaps to allow subsequent excimer laser ablation. The initial high-energy, low pulse femtolaser systems have evolved to present day low energy, high-pulse systems with enhanced precision and minimum collateral damage. The most recent innovation of flapless intrastromal lenticule extraction has marked a significant leap forward, with the elimination of flap-related complications, improved biomechanical stability and a better-preserved ocular surface. With further technological advancements, the refractive applications of this procedure will expand to encompass all types of refractive error with minimum complications and optimal outcomes.

REFERENCES

1. Meyer-Schwickerath G. Light Coagulation. St. Louis, Missouri: CV Mosby Company; 1960.
2. Palanker DV, Blumenkranz MS, Marmor MF. Fifty years of ophthalmic laser therapy. Arch Ophthalmol. 2011;129:1613-9.
3. Schawlow AL, Townes CH. Infrared and optical masers. Phys Rev.1958;112(6): 1940-9.
4. Maiman TH. Stimulated optical radiation in ruby. Nature. 1960;187:493-4.
5. Zaret MM, Breinin GM, Schmidt H, et al. Ocular lesions produced by an optical maser (laser). Science. 1961;134:1525-6.
6. Bridges WB. Laser oscillation in singly ionized argon in visible spectrum. Appl Phys Lett. 1964;4:128.
7. Krueger RR, Rabinowitz YS, Binder PS. The 25th anniversary of excimer lasers in refractive surgery: historical review. J Refract Surg. 2010;26(10):749-60.
8. Bahrawy ME, Alió JL. Excimer laser 6th generation: state of the art and refractive surgical outcomes. Eye Vis (Lond). 2015;2:6.
9. Belin, MW. Evaluating Emerging Refractive Technologies. Int Ophthalmol Clin. 2002;42:1-18.
10. Sato T, Akiyama K, Shibata H. A new surgical approach to myopia. Am J Ophthalmol. 1953;36:823-9.
11. Barraquer JI. Queratomileusis para la corrección de la miopía. Arch Soc Amer Oftal Optom. 1964;5:27.
12. Swinger CA, Krumeich J, Cassiday D. Planar lamellar refractive keratoplasty. J Refract Surg. 1986;2:17.
13. Ruiz LA, Rowsej JJ. In situ keratomileusis. Invest Ophthalmol Vis Sci. 1988;29:392.
14. Reinstein DZ, Archer TJ, Gobbe M. The history of LASIK. J Refract Surg. 2012;28(4):291-8.
15. Srinivasan R, Wynne JJ, Blum SE. Far-UV photoetching of organic material. Laser Focus. 1983:62-66.
16. Cotliar AM, Schubert HD, Mandel ER, et al. Excimer laser radial keratotomy. Ophthalmology. 1985;92(2):206-8.
17. Marshall J, Trokel S, Rothery S, et al. An ultrastructural study of corneal incisions induced by an excimer laser at 193 nm. Ophthalmology. 1985;92(6):749-58.
18. McDonald MB, Liu JC, Byrd TJ, et al. Central photorefractive keratectomy for myopia: Partially sighted and normally sighted eyes. Ophthalmology. 1991;98:1327-38.
19. Pallikaris IG, Papatzanaki ME, Siganos DS, et al. A corneal flap technique for laser in situ keratomileusis—Human studies. Arch Ophthalmol. 1991;109(12):1699-1702.
20. Ito M, Quantock AJ, Malhan S, et al. Picosecond laser in situ keratomileusis with a 1053-nm Nd:YLF laser. J Refract Surg. 1996;12(6):721-8.
21. Krueger RR, Juhasz T, Gualano A, et al. The picosecond laser for nonmechanical laser in situ keratomileusis. J Refract Surg. 1998;14(4):467-9.
22. Krueger RR, Quantock AJ, Juhasz T, et al. Ultrastructure of picosecond laser intrastromal photodisruption. J Refract Surg. 1996;12(5):607-12.

23. Stern D, Schoenlein RW, Puliafito CA, et al. Corneal ablation by nanosecond, picosecond, and femtosecond lasers at 532 and 625 nm. Arch Ophthalmol. 1989;107(4):587-92.
24. Kurtz RM, Horvath C, Liu HH, et al. Lamellar refractive surgery with scanned intrastromal picosecond and femtosecond laser pulses in animal eyes. J Refract Surg. 1998;14(5):541-8.
25. Juhasz T, Loesel FH, Kurtz RM, et al. Corneal refractive surgery with femtosecond lasers. IEEE J Select Topics Quantum Electron. 1999;5:902-10.
26. Hjortdal J, Nielsen E, Vestergaard A, et al. Inverse cutting of posterior lamellar corneal grafts by a femtosecond laser. Open Ophthalmol J. 2012;6:19-22.
27. Callou TP, Garcia R, Mukai A, et al. Advances in femtosecond laser technology. Clin Ophthalmol. 2016;10:697-703.
28. Lubatschowski H, Maatz G, Heisterkamp U, et al. Application of ultrashort laser pulses for intrastromal refractive surgery. Graefe' Arch Clin Exp Ophthalmol. 2000;238:33-9.
29. Heisterkamp A, Mamom T, Drommer W, et al. Photodisruption with ultrashort laser pulses for intrastromal refractive surgery. Laser Phys. 2003;13(5):743-8.
30. Ratkay-Traub I, Ferincz IE, Juhasz T, et al. First clinical results with the femtosecond neodynium-glass laser in refractive surgery. J Refract Surg. 2003;19(2):94-103.
31. Sekundo W, Kunert K, Russmann CH, et al. First efficacy and safety study of femtosecond lenticule extraction for the correction of myopia. J Cataract Refract Surg. 2008;34:1513-20.
32. Blum M, Kunert KS, Engelbrecht C, et al. Femtosecond lenticule extraction (FLEx) - Results after 12 months in myopic astigmatism. Klin Monbl Augenheilkd. 2010;227:961-5.
33. Sekundo W, Kunert KS, Blum M. Small incision corneal refractive surgery using the small incision lenticule extraction (SMILE) procedure for the correction of myopia and myopic astigmatism: results of a 6-month prospective study. Br J Ophthalmol. 2011;95(3):335-9.

Chapter

2

Patient Counseling and Preoperative Evaluation

Sridevi Nair, Manpreet Kaur, Jeewan S Titiyal

INTRODUCTION

Small incision lenticule extraction (SMILE) is a relatively recent addition to the world of refractive surgery and emerging as a safe and successful alternative to femtosecond laser-assisted in situ keratomileusis (FS-LASIK) for the correction of refractive error. It is comparable to FS-LASIK in terms of safety, efficacy and predictability of refractive error correction in myopia and myopic astigmatism. Comprehensive patient evaluation and preoperative counseling help achieve optimal outcomes while maximizing patient satisfaction. The following chapter elucidates the important points one needs to keep in mind before planning a patient for SMILE.[1]

CLINICAL HISTORY

The detailed clinical history is pertinent for the correct planning of a refractive surgery. Before proceeding to ocular history, one should embark on taking a detailed *medical and social history* (Table 2.1).[2]

Table 2.1: Salient points of history taking in a patient planned to undergo small incision lenticule extraction (SMILE)

Ocular history	*Systemic and social history*
▪ Refractive stability: Last change of glasses	▪ Age >21 years
▪ Past history of ocular herpes infection	▪ History of keloid formation
▪ Strabismus	▪ Any past or current autoimmune diseases
▪ Past refractive surgery	▪ Chronic intake of medications
▪ Past history of any other ocular surgery	▪ Past history of diabetes mellitus
▪ Contact lens use/any intolerance	▪ Occupational history: Involved in contact sports, martial arts, armed forces, etc.
▪ History of ocular allergies, dry eye	▪ Pregnancy or breastfeeding
▪ Family history of keratoconus	

Small incision lenticule extraction is Food and Drug Administration (FDA) approved for patients whose age is more than 21 years, as patients younger than this may not have attained refractive stability. Patients nearing presbyopic age may not be good candidates either as they would still require glasses for near activities after surgery. These patients also have a higher risk of developing a visually significant cataract as they age further. Patients in the presbyopic age group should be explained that although before the refractive surgery they may not have required glasses for near work (due to the myopia), this advantage may be lost post-surgery once they are emmetropic.

Occupational history: The nature of the patient's occupation and social history is important, as those involved in contact sports, martial arts or the armed forces may particularly benefit from SMILE as compared to LASIK or femtosecond refractive lenticule extraction (FLEx), due to the avoidance of a flap and the subsequent risk of a traumatic flap dislocation. However, one should also take into account the restrictions placed on the minimum uncorrected visual acuity (UCVA) or best-corrected visual acuity (BCVA) they need to have or the type of refractive surgery they are allowed to undergo by their prospective employers.

Systemic history: The major systemic contraindications to performing SMILE are similar to those applied to LASIK screening. These are mostly conditions that affect corneal wound healing after laser refractive surgery. As per the FDA guidelines, patients suffering from the following *systemic conditions* are *not good candidates* for undergoing laser vision correction:[3]

- *Diabetes mellitus:* It is associated with a number of factors like increased risk for postoperative infections, poor epithelial healing postoperatively and increased propensity to develop a cataract later on. All of these may adversely affect the visual outcomes of refractive surgery. Well-controlled diabetes is a relative contraindication, while uncontrolled diabetes is an absolute contraindication for surgery.
- Systemic diseases leading to *immune-deficient states,* such as acquired immunodeficiency syndrome (AIDS) and systemic malignancies, are a relative contraindication to SMILE as they may make the patient more prone to postoperative infections.
- *Pregnant or breastfeeding women* are absolutely contraindicated for undergoing SMILE as these patients tend to show refractive instability, changes in corneal hydration status and an increased risk for post-operative ectasia. They are at a higher risk of being under or over-corrected by laser refractive surgery due to the abnormal corneal healing process and the refractive instability.
- Patients with a propensity to develop dermatological keloids may show abnormal corneal wound healing, due to which most clinicians treat this as a relative contraindication for surgery.

Medication history: Patients taking certain medications like isotretinoin (used for treatment of acne vulgaris) and antihistamines may experience symptoms of dry eye disease or an exacerbation of preexisting dry eye disease. This could in turn adversely affect epithelial healing after surgery. Other medications interfering with corneal wound healing include drugs such as amiodarone, sumatriptan or hormone replacement therapy.[3,4]

Ocular history: The following *ocular history* should be probed into and patients with conditions described below are *not suitable candidates* for SMILE.

- *Refractive error*: Patients with an unstable refraction, showing changes of 0.5 D or more in the past one year are not ideal candidates for undergoing SMILE. Stable manifest refraction over the past year as demonstrated by a change of less than 0.50 D manifest refraction spherical equivalent (MRSE) is required.
- History of *ocular ectatic diseases* like keratoconus and pellucid marginal degeneration (PMD) are an absolute contraindication for undergoing SMILE as these patients are at a high-risk of post SMILE ectasia. Family history for such conditions should also be probed into and documented.
- Patients with history of uncontrolled *ocular allergic disease* associated with eye rubbing or history of other external disease like blepharitis should be evaluated for the presence of active disease on clinical examination before being planned for surgery.
- A history of past ocular *herpes infection* forms a relative contraindication for SMILE. Such patients should be made aware of the increased risk of recurrent herpetic disease after surgery.
- Patients with a history of other ocular pathologies like glaucoma, uveitis and retinal tears or detachment are not suitable to undergo refractive surgeries.
- Patients who are using contact lenses should be advised to discontinue them before surgery. Soft contact lens use should be discontinued for at least 2 weeks and rigid gas permeables (RGPs) should be discontinued for at least 3–4 weeks before surgery.
- Patients with a known history of significant dry eye disease or other ocular surface disease like epithelial basement membrane dystrophy (EBMD) are not well-suited for SMILE.
- Patients with history of poor vision in one eye (or one-eyed patients) should be discouraged from undergoing an elective refractive surgery in the only seeing eye. They should be clearly explained the possible vision threatening complications associated with surgery, even though their incidence might be very low.
- Patients with a past history of strabismus should be warned about the possibility of a recurrence of deviation after the refractive surgery. Also, the strabismus surgery if required should ideally be performed before the refractive procedure.

CLINICAL EXAMINATION

A detailed systemic as well as clinical ocular examination along with investigations including contrast testing, corneal topography, tomography and aberrometry should be performed (Box 2.1).

Systemic Examination

An important part of examination comprises of assessing the patients' general demeanor. An excessively anxious patient may have trouble in lying still or following surgeon's instructions during the surgical procedure.

Patients suffering from any musculoskeletal condition such as *kyphosis or scoliosis,* which prevents them from lying down straight during the surgery, are not candidates for SMILE.

Presence of collagen vascular diseases, pregnancy, breastfeeding, immunodeficiencies and uncontrolled diabetes mellitus are also contraindications for SMILE.

Box 2.1: Comprehensive ocular examination of a patient planned to undergo small incision lenticule extraction

- Gross clinical exam
  - Deep set eyes/small palpebral fissure
- Refraction: Manifest and cycloplegic: Up to –8 D myopia, up to –0.5 D cylinder
- Visual acuity: UCVA and BCVA
- Detailed slit-lamp examination
  - External surface/lid examination
  - Corneal scars
  - Corneal thinning/ectatic changes
  - Endothelial pathologies
- Ocular surface examination: Schirmer's I test, TBUT
- Pupillary examination: Mesopic pupil <8 mm
- Fundus examination: Periphery screening—rule out pathological lesions
- Tonometry
- Corneal pachymetry: Corneal thickness <480 microns or a residual stromal bed thickness (RSBT) <250 microns unsuitable
- Endothelial cell count
- Determining ocular dominance
- Corneal topography
- Contrast sensitivity
- Aberrometry: Increased HOAs present preoperatively may affect postoperative patient visual satisfaction

(UCVA: Uncorrected visual acuity; BCVA: Best-corrected visual acuity; TBUT: Tear-film breakup time; HOAs: Higher-order aberrations).

Ocular Examination

Ocular Adnexal Examination

In patients with very *deep set eyes* or *extremely small palpebral fissures,* docking would be more challenging. Such eyes are also more prone to suction loss during the procedure. Patient with conditions resulting in *frequent squeezing of lids* (like blepharospasm) or *excessive tearing* also pose a difficulty during the above steps. Suction loss is a common complication seen with SMILE. The reasons for this include relatively longer suction time needed in SMILE (25–35 seconds) and the fact that SMILE is a low pressure system (about 35 mm Hg). Therefore, these patients might pose a challenge during the surgery.[5]

Ocular Motility Assessment

Ocular motility examination is required to detect and evaluate any manifest or latent deviation, which may become manifest post surgery.

Visual Acuity

Uncorrected distance visual acuity and BCVA should be documented.

Refraction

Both objective (especially in hypermetropes) and subjective refraction should be performed. Determination of the vertex distance is important as the laser correction is made at the corneal level. The present FDA-approved indications include:

- Reduction or elimination of myopia ≥ –1.00 D to ≤ –8.00 D with ≤ –0.50 D cylinder
- MRSE ≤ –8.25 D in the eye to be treated.

SMILE is not FDA approved, at present, for treating astigmatism and hyperopia. However, FDA trials are underway to assess the safety and efficacy of SMILE in up to 10 D of myopia and 3 D of astigmatism. A trial is also recruiting patients for hyperopic correction using SMILE for an error up to 7 D.

Contrast Sensitivity

Contrast sensitivity (CS) has been shown to reduce postoperatively after LASIK and photorefractive keratectomy (PRK). Recent studies have shown similar reduction post SMILE too, though less than that seen post LASIK. Though CS usually recovers within the first year post surgery, patients with decreased preoperative contrast should be explained about this possible after effect.[6,7]

Slit-lamp Examination

A comprehensive slit-lamp examination is essential to rule out conditions which may adversely impact the postoperative outcome. Eyelid pathologies like blepharitis and meibomian gland disease need to be satisfactorily treated before surgery. Patients with active ocular allergic diseases should not undergo SMILE until their disease has been controlled with treatment. Patients with features of EBMD, other stromal dystrophies, and stromal scars are not good candidates for SMILE. Signs suggestive of ectasia, such as corneal thinning or steepening should be looked for, as it is not advisable to perform SMILE in conditions like keratoconus or PMD. Patients with other vision limiting conditions like corneal edema, corneal guttata and signs suggestive of Fuchs' endothelial dystrophy should not be planned for SMILE. Patients with lenticular opacities or cataract should be explained that they may not benefit much from a corneal refractive surgery and thus are not good candidates for surgery.

Ocular Surface Examination for Dry Eye Syndrome

The ocular surface and tear film health should be evaluated to rule out ocular surface diseases like dry eyes. Refractive surgeries like LASIK and SMILE are associated with the development of postoperative dry eye disease and decrease in corneal sensitivity. Thus, preoperative dry eye disease is a contraindication for performing SMILE till the disease activity has been adequately controlled on therapy. Patients with severe active dry eye disease should be advised against any type of cornea-based refractive surgery. Well-controlled, mild-moderate dry eye disease is also a relative contraindication for SMILE.[8-10]

Pupillary Examination

The measurement of preoperative pupillary diameter in dim light conditions is crucial, as a pupillary diameter which is greater than the optical zone may result in increased ocular aberrations (especially spherical aberrations) in the postoperative period. This may lead to disturbing symptoms like glare and haloes in the patient. Patients with a mesopic pupil size greater than 8 mm are not good candidates for surgery.[11]

Fundus Examination

A dilated fundus examination to rule out any retinal pathology is imperative as many patients undergoing SMILE may have high myopia, which in itself places them at a higher risk for retinal tears and detachment. Patients with peripheral retinal lesions like lattices, holes, etc. should be treated for the same before proceeding with refractive surgery.

Tonometry

Preoperative intraocular pressure (IOP) should be documented to rule out ocular hypertension or glaucoma. Postoperative IOP should be noted with caution as corneal thinning after SMILE may give falsely low readings.

INVESTIGATIONS

- *Corneal Topography:* The screening criteria applied to detect at risk or ectatic cornea in patients undergoing SMILE is similar to that applied in LASIK patients. SMILE is contraindicated in keratoconus patients and keratoconus suspects. The underlying hypothesis behind the theoretical biomechanical superiority of SMILE over LASIK should be interpreted only in normal corneas with no other suspicious signs of ectasia.[12]

  A number of corneal topographic parameters and features help identify the patient with a normal, suspicious or abnormal cornea, preoperatively. Postoperative corneal ectasia is a dreaded complication that may be seen after any corneal refractive surgery including SMILE. Different modalities like slit-scanning videokeratography, Scheimpflug camera devices, and wavefront analysis have been used to identify these patterns. Scoring systems like ectasia risk score system (ERSS) (proposed by Randleman et al.) have been used to stratify patients into different risk categories for development of postoperative ectasia according to the number and severity of the preoperative parameters. Topographic features like inferior elevation, steeper inferior curvature, excessive thinning of the steepest zone and a skewed astigmatic axis without the normal bowtie pattern are suspicious of keratoconus. The more recent parameters studied on the Pentacam include Belin-Ambrósio Enhanced Ectasia Display (BAD), Ambrósio Relational Thickness (ART), calculated as the thinnest pachymetric value divided by the minimal (ART-Min), maximal (ART-Max) and average (ART-Mid) meridians of pachymetric progression and the D-value calculated to provide optimal sensitivity and specificity.[13,14]
- *Corneal Pachymetry:* Patients with corneal thickness less than 480 microns or a residual stromal bed thickness (RSBT) less than 250 microns are not suitable for SMILE. The RSBT in SMILE is calculated as the stromal thickness below the posterior lenticule interface plus the stromal component of the overlying cap between the anterior lenticule interface and the epithelium. Percentage tissue altered (PTA) is a new metric term that has been recently introduced, and is deemed to result in an increased risk of ectasia if its value is more than 40%. For SMILE, PTA is calculated as:

  PTA = (Lenticule thickness + Cap thickness)/CCT.

  This cut-off of PTA requiring to be less than 40% is applicable to normal corneas only. In the presence of topographic abnormalities, the maximal safe limit for PTA would be much lower.[15,16]

- *Wavefront testing/aberrometry:* Preoperative aberrometry can aid in detecting patients with increased ocular aberrations. This is significant as ocular aberrations have been found to further increase after refractive surgeries. Though both FS-LASIK and SMILE lead to increased ocular aberrations, the aberrations induced are less post SMILE. Wavefront-guided LASIK, however, has been found to be comparable to SMILE in terms of aberrations induced.[17]

DECISION-MAKING AND CASE SELECTION

Careful case selection is essential to avoid unhappy and dissatisfied patients in the postoperative period. A comprehensive workup will help to rule out the cases not suitable to undergo refractive surgery. However, even in cases presumed fit to undergo refractive surgery, the choice of the refractive procedure may vary from one patient to another. Certain patient characteristics may make them unsuitable for a specific refractive surgery, and preoperative identification of such factors will help achieve optimal visual and anatomical outcomes as well as patient satisfaction. The absolute and relative contraindications for SMILE are summarized in Table 2.2. Factors affecting decision-making and case selection are discussed below and summarized in Table 2.3.

Table 2.2: Absolute and relative contraindications for small incision lenticule extraction (SMILE)

Absolute contraindications to SMILE	*Relative contraindications to SMILE*
Corneal ectatic disorders like keratoconus, pellucid marginal degeneration	Age <21 years
Unstable refractive error	Mild/treated dry eye
Pregnant or breastfeeding	Past ocular herpes infection
Active uncontrolled ocular allergy, severe dry eye, blepharitis	Immunodeficient states
Uncontrolled glaucoma, uveitis	Diabetes mellitus (controlled)
One eyed/single eyed functional status	Epithelial basement membrane dystrophy
Exposure keratopathy	History of keloid formation
	Autoimmune disorders

Table 2.3: Patient selection criteria for decision-making before refractive surgery

Cases where SMILE scores over LASIK	*Cases where LASIK scores over SMILE*
Mild ocular surface disease	Hyperopia
Higher refractive error	Astigmatism
Contact sports, martial arts, military personnel	Post refractive surgery enhancement

(LASIK: Laser-assisted in situ keratomileusis; SMILE: Small incision lenticule extraction).

Situations when SMILE may Have an Edge

- SMILE is a third generation laser refractive surgical procedure developed as an advancement over the femtosecond LASIK and FLEx. Recent studies have found SMILE to offer advantages over LASIK and PRK in certain groups of patients. SMILE is associated with a lower risk and severity of postoperative dry eyes as compared to other refractive surgeries. The corneal sensitivity is better maintained after surgery. The reason for this could be both lesser damage to subbasal nerves due to the smaller penetrating tunnel (about 40–60° arc) than LASIK (300° arc) and faster recovery of corneal innervation postoperatively. This property may make it a better choice for patients who have mild *ocular surface disorders* preoperatively, but are motivated to undergo a refractive procedure.[8-10]
- For the correction of the same refractive error, a cornea undergoing SMILE is associated with a better mechanical stability postoperatively than that seen after LASIK. SMILE also involves tissue subtraction rather than ablative tissue destruction as seen in LASIK. This may make it a better option for *patients requiring higher refractive error correction.*[18] However, at present, SMILE has received FDA approval for correction of MRSE less than or equal to –8.25 D. It has received CE approval for correction of MRSE less than or equal to 11.5 D, though FDA trials for the same are underway.
- SMILE being a flapless procedure is free of the flap-related complications such as buttonholing, free cap, flap tears and traumatic avulsion. This makes it a preferred procedure for *patients prone to traumatic dislocation of the flaps*, like those involved in contact sports, martial arts and military services.
- Studies have observed SMILE to induce less higher-order aberrations (HOAs) than traditional femtosecond LASIK. HOAs could result in symptoms such as glare and halos. SMILE has been found to induce lesser spherical aberrations, which may be particularly advantageous in *patients with larger pupils*, as these patients tend to have more pronounced symptoms due to increased spherical aberrations.[7,11]

Situations when SMILE is not the Best Option

Though SMILE has been found to have a number of advantageous features over LASIK, there are certain situations where patients may do better with a LASIK than SMILE.

- Patients with *deep set eyes, small palpebral fissures, those too anxious or unable to follow instructions* or squeezing the eye too much are more prone to suction loss during the surgery. Suction loss might be more commonly seen in SMILE than LASIK. The reasons for this include longer suction time needed in SMILE (25–35 seconds) than that needed in femtosecond

LASIK (femtosecond part of the procedure lasts for 18–20 seconds only) and the fact that SMILE is a low pressure system (about 35 mm Hg). Thus, patients prone to suction loss should be given the option of femtosecond LASIK or PRK.[5]

- Though studies are underway, SMILE is not an established procedure for performing *hyperopic refractive correction*. Also, notable under-correction was seen when it was used to treat higher amounts of *astigmatism*. SMILE is not yet FDA approved for treating hyperopia or astigmatism more than 0.5 D. These patients may be candidates for LASIK or PRK rather than SMILE.[19,20]
- Though a number of methods like FS-LASIK and PRK have been tried for *post-SMILE enhancement* and retreatment, at present, there is no established protocol for performing repeat SMILE. Also, SMILE has a relatively steep learning curve and may be more challenging to perform than LASIK in the initial phase of learning for the operating surgeon, adversely affecting the outcomes.[21,22]

PATIENT COUNSELING AND INFORMED CONSENT

Proper patient counseling is an important step in ensuring good results after any refractive surgery. The surgeon should assess the patient's expectations before deciding for the surgery. Unrealistic expectations like an improvement beyond the BCVA or perfect vision after refractive surgery should be dealt with appropriately. The patient should be informed about the options available to correct the refractive error (suitable for his/her clinical profile) and explained the advantages and disadvantages of each in detail. Patients nearing presbyopic age should be explained that the treatment is not aimed at tackling presbyopia and that they would require glasses for near once presbyopia sets in. They should also be explained in detail about the possible complications, delay in visual recovery, residual refractive errors and need for enhancements.

The patient should be explained about the steps of surgery, duration of each step, possible complications and expected visual outcomes of the surgery. Additionally, the patient should be explained of what he is expected to do during surgery, as described below.

- The patient should be able to lie down flat during the whole duration of the procedure.
- The patient should be able to continuously fixate at a blinking light during the surgical procedure.
- He should be able to follow surgeon's instructions and should avoid moving or squeezing his lids during the surgery.

An informed consent should be obtained before the surgery by the operating surgeon. A few points to keep in mind are as follows:

- A detailed discussion of the patient's clinical findings in a lucid language understandable to the patient is required.
- He should be made aware of the different surgical options at his disposal along with the advantages and disadvantages of each.
- The patient should be given ample opportunity to ask questions and clear doubts regarding the surgery's expected outcomes.
- The patient should be made aware of the pros and cons of the surgery, and explained the possibility of occurrence of post-surgical complications and their potential implications.
- The consent should have been read and understood by the patient before he signs it, ideally a day before the surgery. The patient should not be sedated or have pupils dilated while doing so.

CONCLUSION

Comprehensive preoperative workup including a detailed history as well as thorough ocular examination is essential to identify patients unsuitable for refractive surgery. Preoperative counseling to address unrealistic patient expectations and give them an overview of the surgical procedure with its pros and cons go a long way in ensuring a satisfied patient as well as a happy surgeon.

REFERENCES

1. Shen Z, Shi K, Yu Y, et al. Small incision lenticule extraction (SMILE) versus femtosecond laser-assisted in situ keratomileusis (FS-LASIK) for myopia: a systematic review and meta-analysis. PLoS One. 2016;11(7):e0158176.
2. American Academy of Ophthalmology. (2008). Summary recommendations for keratorefractive laser surgery. [online] Available from https://www.aao.org/clinical-statement/summary-recommendations-lasik--january-2008. [Accessed July 2017]
3. AlKharashi M, Bower KS, Stark WJ, et al. Refractive Surgery in Systemic and Autoimmune Disease. Middle East Afr J Ophthalmol. 2014;21(1):18-24.
4. Miles S, McGlathery W, Abernathie B. The importance of screening for laser-assisted in situ keratomileusis operation (LASIK) before prescribing isotretinoin. J Am Acad Dermatol. 2006;54(1):180-1.
5. Wong CW, Chan C, Tan D, et al. Incidence and management of suction loss in refractive lenticule extraction. J Cataract Refract Surg. 2014;40(12):2002-10.
6. Sekundo W, Gertnere J, Bertelmann T, et al. One-year refractive results, contrast sensitivity, high-order aberrations and complications after myopic small-incision lenticule extraction (ReLEx SMILE). Graefes Arch Clin Exp Ophthalmol. 2014;252(5):837-43.
7. Ganesh S, Batra A. Comparative study of visual outcome between femtosecond lasik with excimer laser and all femtosecond ReLex small incision lenticule extraction (smile). IOSR J Dent Med Sci. 2015;14(11):44-53.
8. Denoyer A, Landman E, Trinh L, et al. Dry eye disease after refractive surgery: comparative outcomes of small incision lenticule extraction versus LASIK. Ophthalmology. 2015;122(4):669-76.

9. Li M, Zhao J, Shen Y, et al. Comparison of dry eye and corneal sensitivity between small incision lenticule extraction and femtosecond LASIK for myopia. PLoS One. 2013;8(10):e77797.
10. Xu Y, Yang Y. Dry eye after small incision lenticule extraction and LASIK for myopia. J Refract Surg. 2014;30:186-90.
11. Lin F, Xu Y, Yang Y. Comparison of the visual results after SMILE and femtosecond laser-assisted LASIK for myopia. J Refract Surg. 2014;20:248-54.
12. Randleman JB. Ectasia after corneal refractive surgery: nothing to SMILE about. J Refract Surg. 2016;32(7):434-5.
13. Ambrósio R Jr, Caiado AL, Guerra FP, et al. Novel pachymetric parameters based on corneal tomography for diagnosing keratoconus. J Refract Surg. 2011;27(10):753-8.
14. Hashemi H, Beiranvand A, Yekta A, et al. Pentacam top indices for diagnosing subclinical and definite keratoconus. J Curr Ophthalmol. 2016;28(1):21-6.
15. Santhiago MR. Percent tissue altered and corneal ectasia. Curr Opin Ophthalmol. 2016;27(4):311-5.
16. El-Naggar MT. Bilateral ectasia after femtosecond laser-assisted small-incision lenticule extraction. J Cataract Refract Surg. 2015;41:884-8.
17. Chen X, Wang Y, Zhang J, et al. Comparison of ocular higher-order aberrations after SMILE and wavefront-guided femtosecond LASIK for myopia. BMC Ophthalmol. 2017;17:42.
18. Wu D, Wang Y, Zhang L, et al. Corneal biomechanical effects: small-incision lenticule extraction versus femtosecond laser–assisted laser in situ keratomileusis. J Cataract Refract Surg. 2014;40:954-96.
19. Moshirfar M, McCaughey MV, Reinstein DZ, et al. Small-incision lenticule extraction. J Cataract Refract Surg. 2015;41(3):652-65.
20. Ivarsen A, Hjortdal J. Correction of myopic astigmatism with small incision lenticule extraction. J Refract Surg. 2014;30:240-7.
21. Vestergaard AH. Past and present of corneal refractive surgery; a retrospective study of long-term results after photorefractive keratectomy, and a prospective study of refractive lenticule extraction. Acta Ophthalmol. 2014;92:1-21.
22. Riau AK, Ang HP, Lwin NC, et al. Comparison of four different VisuMax circle patterns for flap creation after small incision lenticule extraction. J Refract Surg. 2013;29:236-44.

Chapter 3

Corneal Wound Healing, Morphological and Biomechanical Changes after Small Incision Lenticule Extraction

Pranita Sahay, Manpreet Kaur, Anand Singh Brar, Jeewan S Titiyal

INTRODUCTION

Postoperative corneal wound healing and biomechanical remodeling play a significant role in determining the visual outcome and biomechanical stability after corneal refractive surgeries. An altered wound healing response may lead to undercorrection, overcorrection, regression or irregular astigmatism, and result in suboptimal visual outcomes. Moreover, corneal haze and epithelial ingrowth may be observed as a result of the variable biological response during the process of wound remodeling.[1] The corneal epithelium, stromal keratocytes, nerve fibers, inflammatory cells, and lacrimal glands are involved in the biomechanical remodeling after refractive surgery, and their in-depth understanding is essential to achieve optimal refractive and physiological outcomes (Table 3.1).

CORNEAL WOUND HEALING CASCADE

The phenomenon of corneal wound healing encompasses a complex cascade of events that is initiated in response to corneal trauma (Flowchart 3.1). The femtosecond (FS) laser-induced insult to the corneal stroma in small incision lenticule extraction (SMILE) stimulates the release of various cytokines, chemokines, and growth factors from the corneal epithelium as well as keratocytes, such as interleukin-1 (IL-1), tumor necrosis factor-alpha (TNF-α), epidermal growth factor (EGF), and platelet-derived growth factor (PDGF).[1-5] This results in the apoptosis of keratocytes and incites further release of inflammatory mediators. Few keratocytes also undergo necrosis and stimulate the proliferation of inflammatory cells like monocytes, granulocytes, and lymphocytes in that region. These inflammatory cells phagocytose the necrotic and apoptotic cell debris and further amplify the inflammatory response by release of various mediators. The remaining keratocytes in the surrounding stroma are activated and transform into fibroblasts and myofibroblasts. These transformed cells migrate to the cell-depleted

Table 3.1: Morphological, biomechanical, biochemical, and functional changes after small incision lenticule extraction (SMILE)

Parameter	Changes after SMILE
Morphological changes	Corneal nerve fiber layer ▪ Reduction in sub-basal nerve length and density (SLD) • Relative preservation of central sub-basal nerve density • Recovery of the SLD to the preoperative level by 6–12 months Corneal keratocyte density ▪ Keratocyte apoptosis and decreased density: Do not recover ▪ Surrounding keratocyte activation: Increased interface activation on confocal microscopy
Biomechanical changes	▪ Better biomechanical strength after SMILE: Preservation of anterior stromal fibers which have greater tensile strength than posterior stromal fibers ▪ Decrease in corneal hysteresis (CH) and corneal resistance factor (CRF) on ORA ▪ Decrease in applanation time and deformation amplitude on Corvis ST
Inflammatory mediators	▪ Elevated levels of nerve growth factor (NGF), interleukins (IL-1α and IL-6), transforming growth factor beta1 (TGF-β1) ▪ No change in levels of tumor necrosis factor-alpha (TNF-α), matrix metalloproteinases (MMP-9), intercellular adhesion molecule-1 (ICAM-1), and interferons (IFN-γ) ▪ Increased levels of CD11b, HSP-47, and fibronectin
Functional changes	Corneal sensation ▪ Corneal sensation reduced, early recovery as compared to LASIK • Central corneal sensation relatively preserved, better than LASIK ▪ Less risk of postoperative dry eye after SMILE due to better preservation of corneal sensation Ocular surface stability ▪ Decrease in tear meniscus height, TBUT and Schirmer's test values ▪ Increased OSDI score ▪ Increased corneal fluorescein staining

(ORA: Ocular response analyzer; Corvis ST: Corneal visualization Scheimpflug technology; LASIK: Laser-assisted in situ keratomileusis; TBUT: Tear film breakup time; OSDI: Ocular surface disease index).

regions, actively synthesize extracellular matrix including collagen and glycosaminoglycans, release matrix remodeling enzymes such as collagenases and metalloproteinases and result in stromal remodeling.[1-5]

The wound healing response is less exuberant in SMILE as compared to laser-assisted in situ keratomileusis (LASIK), owing to a smaller size of corneal incision and the absence of excimer laser-induced tissue ablation in the former.[2] *Terminal deoxynucleotidyl transferase-mediated dUTP-digoxigenin Nick-End Labeling (TUNEL)* assay is used to detect apoptotic cells after

Flowchart 3.1: Wound healing cascade after small incision lenticule extraction (SMILE).

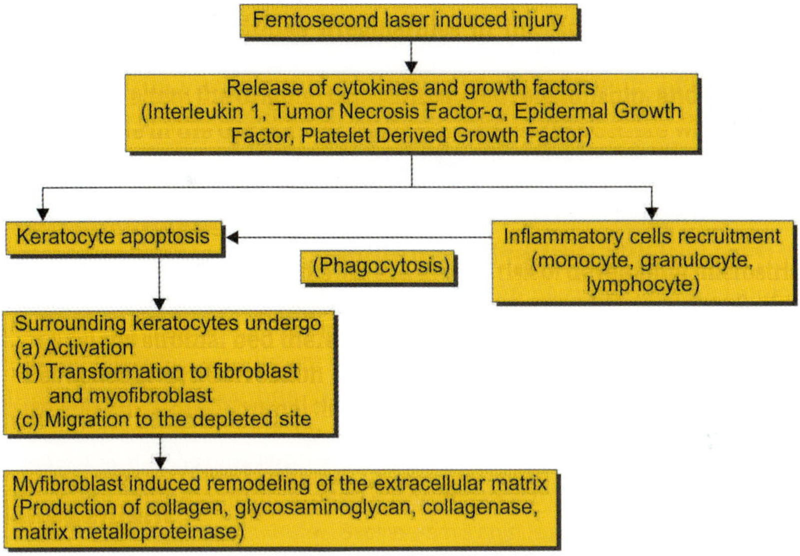

surgery. Apoptosis in the interface region is observed after both LASIK and SMILE, with a peak occurring at 4 hours after the surgery; however, the magnitude of the apoptotic response is much less after SMILE.[2] Immunofluorescence assays have observed a reduced expression of both Ki67, a cell marker of the G1-M phase of mitosis as well as CD11b, a marker of monocytes in SMILE as compared to LASIK.[2]

Wound healing is influenced by the laser energy level, spot sizing, and spacing settings. Unlike other corneal refractive surgeries, the magnitude of refractive error does not influence the postsurgical remodeling in SMILE. This may be explained by the fact that only the shape of the SMILE lenticule changes with the magnitude of refractive error. Increased inflammation is observed with excessive surgical manipulation, such as in thin lenticules (low refractive error) and cases with cap-lenticular adhesions.[6]

MORPHOLOGICAL CHANGES AFTER SMILE

Normal Anatomy of Corneal Nerve Fibers

The cornea receives its sensory innervation from the ophthalmic division of trigeminal nerve via two long ciliary nerves. It divides into multiple branches as it reaches the limbus and anastomizes with the short ciliary nerves before entering the cornea. Together, they constitute both the sensory and autonomic innervation of the cornea. The nerve fibers that enter the cornea at limbus run radially toward the center beneath the anterior one-third of the corneal stroma. In the stroma, these fibers are arranged parallel to the collagen lamella. This gives rise to numerous small fascicules which form the *anterior stromal nerve plexus.* Nerve fibers arising from this anterior stromal plexus then take an abrupt 90° turn and penetrate the bowman's layer (perforation site) to become more superficial. These perforations occur throughout the cornea but are maximally seen in the mid-peripheral areas. Here, they give multiple branches and again take a 90° turn to give rise to the *sub-basal nerve plexus.* Branches from this plexus run obliquely to eventually terminate in the corneal epithelium.

Corneal Nerve Fiber Layer Changes

Confocal microscopy is an in-vivo histological tool that allows the real-time assessment of the corneal architecture, including the nerve plexus and keratocytes. It has been used to evaluate the morphology and regeneration patterns of corneal nerve fibers after SMILE, and a decrease in both the length and density of corneal nerve fibers in the sub-basal plexus has been observed (Figs. 3.1A to F).[7-9] The decrease is most marked after 1 week of surgery, after which the process of nerve regeneration is evident.[7]

The central sub-basal nerve fibers are relatively well preserved after SMILE as compared to FS-LASIK. Li et al. observed the presence of central sub-basal nerves in nearly 100% cases after SMILE at all follow-up visits, in contrast to FS-LASIK wherein less than 30% cases had detectable nerve fibers in the central cornea in the first postoperative month.[7] Immunostaining studies have revealed a faster recovery of stromal nerve fibers after SMILE as compared to LASIK.[7] The rate of regeneration is significantly faster in SMILE till 6 months after surgery, beyond which both procedures exhibit similar corneal innervation. The regenerating nerves are tortuous and thin, and chart their course from the periphery to the center in order to establish a new sub-basal nerve plexus.

The difference in the sub-basal nerve plexus damage and regeneration patterns in SMILE and FS-LASIK is attributed to the incision size. FS-LASIK involves the creation of a lamellar corneal flap which results in the transection of the sub-basal corneal nerve fibers in a circumferential manner, except in the region of the flap hinge. In contrast, the nerve fibers are transected in the small region of the cap side cut (2–5 mm) only during SMILE, thereby resulting in less damage.

Corneal Keratocyte Density

A decrease in keratocyte density has been observed after SMILE as a result of keratocyte necrosis and apoptosis (Figs. 3.2A to C). Both pre-interface and post-interface keratocyte densities are decreased in the immediate postoperative period and do not recover subsequently.[7] Similar persistent decrease in keratocyte density has also been observed after LASIK.[10] The exact clinical significance of stromal keratocytes in preserving a stable ocular surface is largely unknown. However, a strong correlation has been

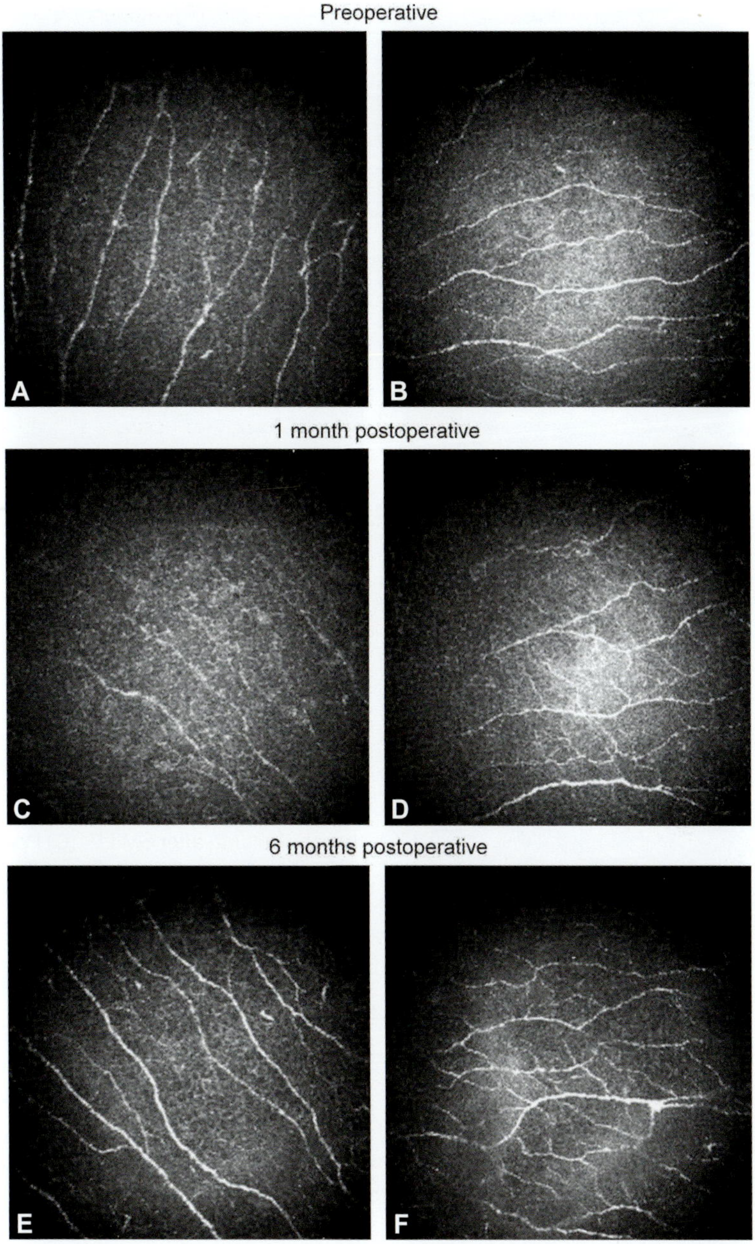

Figs. 3.1A to F: Corneal sub-basal nerve fibers as observed on confocal microscopy before and after small incision lenticule extraction (SMILE). (A and B) Preoperative sub-basal corneal nerve fibers (A: Vertical orientation; B: Horizontal orientation). (C and D) Sub-basal corneal nerve fibers with reduced length and density 1 month after SMILE (C: Vertical orientation; D: Horizontal orientation). Thin and tortuous regenerating nerve fibers are seen. (E and F) Sub-basal corneal nerves 6 months after SMILE (E: Vertical orientation; F: Horizontal orientation). Regeneration is almost complete and the nerve fiber density is similar to the preoperative levels.

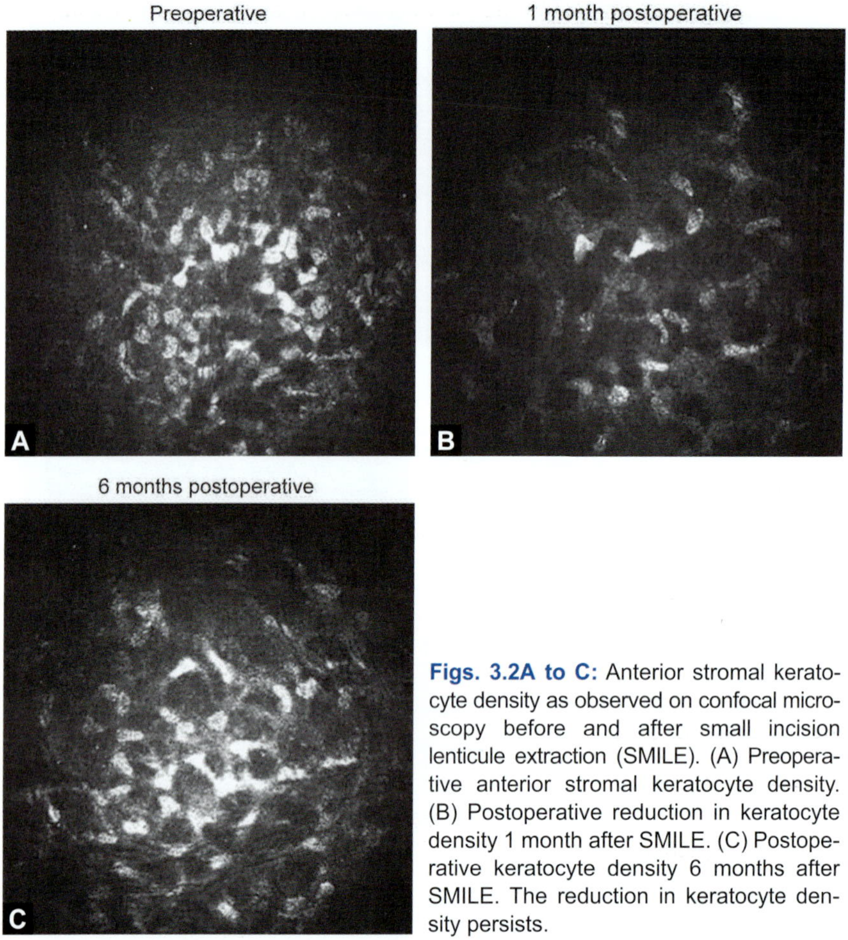

Figs. 3.2A to C: Anterior stromal keratocyte density as observed on confocal microscopy before and after small incision lenticule extraction (SMILE). (A) Preoperative anterior stromal keratocyte density. (B) Postoperative reduction in keratocyte density 1 month after SMILE. (C) Postoperative keratocyte density 6 months after SMILE. The reduction in keratocyte density persists.

observed between the sub-basal nerve density and keratocyte density after both LASIK and photorefractive keratectomy (PRK).[11]

The surrounding keratocytes are activated during the wound healing response observed after SMILE. These activated keratocytes migrate and proliferate to the acellular areas in an attempt to restore the cellular distribution. An increased reflectivity at the interface has been observed during in-vivo confocal microscopy indicating the activated keratocytes.[6] This increased reflectivity is more marked in higher magnitude of refractive errors (–8.00 D), owing to the greater extent of stromal tissue removed.[6]

BIOMECHANICAL CHANGES AFTER SMILE

Corneal biomechanics is a complex interplay of several factors including the external deforming force, the cornea as well as the intraocular pressure (IOP).

It may be defined as the response of corneal tissue to externally applied forces, and is governed by the viscous and elastic properties of the cornea. A decrease in corneal biomechanical stability after various refractive surgical procedures forms the basis of postoperative ectasia. Hence, an in-depth knowledge of the normal anatomy of the corneal stroma and the changes observed after different refractive surgical procedures is essential to determine the safety and stability of the surgery.

Clinical Anatomy

The corneal biomechanical strength depends primarily on the regional variation in the arrangement of stromal collagen fibrils. The corneal stroma consists of around 200 collagen lamellae arranged parallel to each other, with variable levels of interlacing and interlamellar proteoglycan bonds. The anterior stroma has thin, densely packed collagen lamellae, and these branching and interlacing fibers contribute to the main stromal strength.[12] In contrast, the posterior stromal fibers are thicker and sparsely packed, and are less interwoven than the anterior fibers.[13] The anterior stromal strength has been observed to be up to 25% more than that of the posterior stroma.[12,14]

Biomechanical Properties after SMILE

Reinstein et al. proposed a mathematical model to predict the biomechanical strength of the cornea after refractive surgical procedures.[15] As per his model, flap-based procedures result in a vertical transection of the collagen lamellae in the biomechanically strong anterior and peripheral stroma. In contrast, SMILE results in transection of anterior collagen lamellae only in the localized region of cap side cut, thereby preserving the majority of strong anterior and peripheral collagen lamellae after surgery. The refractive lenticule thus extracted consists of relatively weaker collagen fibers of the central stroma, beyond the cap depth of anterior 120 μm. Thus SMILE is postulated to have superior biomechanical stability as compared to conventional flap-based LASIK or surface ablative procedures, and may consequently be more suitable for higher degrees of refractive errors.[15]

Ocular response analyzer (ORA) and Corvis ST (Corneal Visualization Scheimpflug Technology) allow for the objective in-vivo assessment of corneal biomechanics, and have been used in various studies to evaluate the postoperative change in corneal viscosity and elasticity after different refractive surgical procedures.

A decrease in both corneal hysteresis (CH, a measure of corneal viscous damping) and corneal resistance factor (CRF, a measure of corneal viscosity and elasticity) has been documented after SMILE.[16-20] Moreover, a decrease in the deformation amplitude as well as the applanation times has been observed using the Scheimpflug technology of Corvis ST.[16,21]

The decrease in biomechanical strength is less than that compared with flap-based corneal ablative procedures.[16,17] However; the reports are inconsistent, with some studies not observing a difference between SMILE and LASIK, or some studies observing a more significant decrease after LASIK only in higher magnitude of refractive errors (>6.0 D).[18-21]

Posterior corneal elevation is an indicator for development of ectasia, and significantly more increase in posterior elevation is observed after LASIK than after SMILE.[22]

Intraocular pressure is falsely underestimated after corneal refractive surgeries, and this is attributed to the decreased biomechanical strength and increased deformability of the cornea. The IOP measurements are more stable after SMILE, which may indirectly reflect a better biomechanical stability.[23]

INFLAMMATORY MEDIATORS

Various proinflammatory mediators are involved in the process of wound healing after refractive surgery, and they influence the ocular surface stability as well as the development of postoperative dry eye.

Elevated levels of nerve growth factor (NGF), ILs such as IL-1α and IL-6 and transforming growth factor beta1 (TGF-β1) are observed after SMILE. Nerve growth factor is involved in nerve regeneration, IL-1α modulates the function of corneal fibroblasts and TGF-β1 is involved in keratocyte activation, myofibroblast transformation, fibronectin synthesis, and collagen contraction. The increase in the levels of these inflammatory markers is less than flap-based procedures such as LASIK or femtosecond lenticule extraction (FLEx). Moreover, the levels return to the baseline earlier, indicating a faster recovery after SMILE.[6,24,25]

The levels of TNF-α, matrix metalloproteinases (MMP-9), intercellular adhesion molecule-1 (ICAM-1), and interferons (IFN-γ) are not significantly elevated after SMILE, indicating a typically mild inflammatory response.[6,24,25]

Increased levels of CD11b as well as HSP47 are observed after SMILE. CD11b is an inflammatory marker which is expressed on the surface of neutrophils, monocytes, and macrophages, and is mainly localized to the site of side-cut incision. HSP47 is a heat shock protein whose expression is induced in response to cellular stress, and is observed at the site of side cut as well as in the stroma. Fibronectin is secreted by the activated stromal fibroblasts, and its expression correlates with the wound healing response after SMILE.[6]

The inflammatory response is influenced by the surgeon experience and the magnitude of refractive error, and enhanced levels of inflammatory mediators are observed after SMILE during the initial learning curve of the surgeon with low magnitude of refractive errors. Low myopia cases have thinner lenticules, which are associated with difficult dissection and increased intraoperative manipulations, especially where the surgeon itself is in the initial learning stages. This may account for the elevated levels of inflammatory mediators observed in such cases.[6]

The presence and levels of these inflammatory mediators correlate with a decreased ocular surface stability and subjective discomfort as measured by the ocular surface disease index (OSDI).[6,24,25]

FUNCTIONAL CHANGES AFTER SMILE

Maintenance of intact corneal innervations exerts a neurotrophic influence on the ocular surface which is essential to maintain ocular health and stability. Transection of sub-basal corneal nerves leads to a decrease in the central corneal sensations, and subsequently affects the tear secretion, mucin expression as well as the frequency of blinking. All these factors contribute to postoperative dry eye disease and poor ocular health, which is frequently observed after corneal refractive surgeries.

Corneal Sensations

Diminished corneal sensations are observed after SMILE, especially in the central cornea. The corneal sensations begin to recover within the first month of intrastromal refractive surgery, and recover to the preoperative level by 6–12 months.[26-29]

The mean central corneal sensations, though reduced, are better than other corneal ablative procedures, indicating less nerve damage in SMILE. The keratocyte loss after SMILE is less than that in corneal ablative procedures, which is associated with an early recovery of the corneal sensations. SMILE has a major advantage of causing less postoperative dry eye which has been corroborated in various clinical trials.[26-29]

Ocular Surface Stability

Subjective discomfort has been assessed using the OSDI index, and an increase in the OSDI scores is observed after SMILE in the immediate postoperative period. The OSDI score returns to the baseline in a majority of patients by the end of the first postoperative month.

A decrease in postoperative ocular surface stability has been observed after SMILE, in terms of decreased tear breakup time (TBUT) and increased fluorescein (FL) staining of the corneal surface.[26-29]

The OSDI scores, FL staining, and TBUT are less deranged after SMILE than after LASIK, and return to the preoperative levels faster.[26-29]

CONCLUSION

Corneal wound healing plays a major role in determining the postoperative visual outcome, biomechanical strength of the cornea as well as complications after SMILE. Though corneal nerve fiber damage is seen after SMILE, a rapid recovery of the nerve fibers is observed by 3–6 months resulting in better corneal sensations and less risk of postoperative dry eye syndrome. Biomechanical strength of the cornea, though decreased, is thought to be better preserved after SMILE.

REFERENCES

1. Netto MV, Mohan RR, Ambrósio R Jr, et al. Wound healing in the cornea: a review of refractive surgery complications and new prospects for therapy. Cornea. 2005;24(5):509-22.
2. Dong Z, Zhou X, Wu J, et al. Small incision lenticule extraction (SMILE) and femtosecond laser LASIK: comparison of corneal wound healing and inflammation. Br J Ophthalmol. 2014;98(2):263-9.
3. Mohan RR, Mohan RR, Kim WJ, et al. Modulation of TNF-alpha-induced apoptosis in corneal fibroblasts by transcription factor NF-kappaB. Invest Ophthalmol Vis Sci. 2000;41(6):1327-36.
4. Wilson SE, He YG, Weng J, et al. Epithelial injury induces keratocyte apoptosis: hypothesized role for the interleukin-1 system in the modulation of corneal tissue organization and wound healing. Exp Eye Res. 1996;62(4):325-7.
5. Wilson SE, Mohan RR, Mohan RR, et al. The corneal wound healing response: cytokine-mediated interaction of the epithelium, stroma, and inflammatory cells. Prog Retin Eye Res. 2001;20(5):625-37.
6. Liu YC, Teo EP, Lwin NC, et al. Early Corneal Wound Healing and Inflammatory Responses After SMILE: Comparison of the Effects of Different Refractive Corrections and Surgical Experiences. J Refract Surg. 2016;32(5):346-53.
7. Li M, Niu L, Qin B, et al. Confocal comparison of corneal reinnervation after small incision lenticule extraction (SMILE) and femtosecond laser in situ keratomileusis (FS-LASIK). PLoS One. 2013;8(12):e81435.
8. Vestergaard AH, Grønbech KT, Grauslund J, et al. Subbasal nerve morphology, corneal sensation, and tear film evaluation after refractive femtosecond laser lenticule extraction. Graefes Arch Clin Exp Ophthalmol. 2013;251(11):2591-600.
9. Mohamed-Noriega K, Riau AK, Lwin NC, et al. Early corneal nerve damage and recovery following small incision lenticule extraction (SMILE) and laser in situ keratomileusis (LASIK). Invest Ophthalmol Vis Sci. 2014;55(3):1823-34.
10. Erie JC, Nau CB, McLaren JW, et al. Long-term keratocyte deficits in the corneal stroma after LASIK. Ophthalmology. 2004;111(7):1356-61.
11. Lee SJ, Kim JK, Seo KY, et al. Comparison of corneal nerve regeneration and sensitivity between LASIK and laser epithelial keratomileusis (LASEK). Am J Ophthalmol. 2006;141(6):1009-15.
12. Radner W, Zehetmayer M, Aufreiter R, et al. Interlacing and cross-angle distribution of collagen lamellae in the human cornea. Cornea. 1998;17:537-43.
13. Müller LJ, Pels E, Vrensen GF. The specific architecture of the anterior stroma accounts for maintenance of corneal curvature. Br J Ophthalmol. 2001;85(4):437-43.
14. Smolek MK, McCarey BE. Interlamellar adhesive strength in human eyebank corneas. Invest Ophthalmol Vis Sci. 1990;31(6):1087-95.
15. Reinstein DZ, Archer TJ, Randleman JB. Mathematical model to compare the relative tensile strength of the cornea after PRK, LASIK, and small incision lenticule extraction. J Refract Surg. 2013;29(7):454-60.
16. Osman IM, Helaly HA, Abdalla M, et al. Corneal biomechanical changes in eyes with small incision lenticule extraction and laser assisted in situ keratomileusis. BMC Ophthalmol. 2016;16:123.

17. Wu D, Wang Y, Zhang L, et al. Corneal biomechanical effects: small-incision lenticule extraction versus femtosecond laser-assisted laser in situ keratomileusis. J Cataract Refract Surg. 2014;40(6):954-62.
18. Agca A, Ozgurhan EB, Demirok A, et al. Comparison of corneal hysteresis and corneal resistance factor after small incision lenticule extraction and femtosecond laser-assisted LASIK: a prospective fellow eye study. Cont Lens Anterior Eye. 2014;37(2):77-80.
19. Shen Y, Chen Z, Knorz MC, et al. Comparison of corneal deformation parameters after SMILE, LASEK, and femtosecond laser-assisted LASIK. J Refract Surg. 2014;30(5):310-8.
20. Wang D, Liu M, Chen Y, et al. Differences in the corneal biomechanical changes after SMILE and LASIK. J Refract Surg. 2014;30(10):702-7.
21. Sefat SM, Wiltfang R, Bechmann M, et al. Evaluation of Changes in Human Corneas After Femtosecond Laser-Assisted LASIK and Small-Incision Lenticule Extraction (SMILE) Using Non-Contact Tonometry and Ultra-High-Speed Camera (Corvis ST). Curr Eye Res. 2016;41(7):917-22.
22. Wang B, Zhang Z, Naidu RK, et al. Comparison of the change in posterior corneal elevation and corneal biomechanical parameters after small incision lenticule extraction and femtosecond laser-assisted LASIK for high myopia correction. Cont Lens Anterior Eye. 2016;39(3):191-6.
23. Li H, Wang Y, Dou R, et al. Intraocular Pressure Changes and Relationship With Corneal Biomechanics After SMILE and FS-LASIK. Invest Ophthalmol Vis Sci. 2016;57(10):4180-6.
24. Gao S, Li S, Liu L, et al. Early changes in ocular surface and tear inflammatory mediators after small-incision lenticule extraction and femtosecond laser-assisted laser in situ keratomileusis. PLoS One. 2014;9(9):e107370.
25. Zhang C, Ding H, He M, et al. Comparison of Early Changes in Ocular Surface and Inflammatory Mediators between Femtosecond Lenticule Extraction and Small-Incision Lenticule Extraction. PLoS One. 2016;11(3):e0149503.
26. Cai WT, Liu QY, Ren CD, et al. Dry eye and corneal sensitivity after small incision lenticule extraction and femtosecond laser-assisted *in situ* keratomileusis: a Meta-analysis. Int J Ophthalmol. 2017;10(4):632-8.
27. Shen Z, Zhu Y, Song X, et al. Dry Eye after Small Incision Lenticule Extraction (SMILE) versus Femtosecond Laser-Assisted in Situ Keratomileusis (FS-LASIK) for Myopia: A Meta-Analysis. PLoS One. 2016;11(12):e0168081.
28. Denoyer A, Landman E, Trinh L, et al. Dry eye disease after refractive surgery: comparative outcomes of small incision lenticule extraction versus LASIK. Ophthalmology. 2015;122(4):669-76.
29. Li M, Zhao J, Shen Y, et al. Comparison of dry eye and corneal sensitivity between small incision lenticule extraction and femtosecond LASIK for myopia. PLoS One. 2013;8(10):e77797.

Chapter 4

Understanding the Machine and Laser Settings

Anubha Rathi, Manpreet Kaur, Jeewan S Titiyal

INTRODUCTION

The concept of refractive lenticule extraction (ReLEx) heralded a landmark shift in the concept of refractive surgery from the conventional two-step flap-based corneal ablative procedures to a single-step femtosecond laser procedure.[1] The initial procedure involved lifting the flap to extract the refractive lenticule and was known as *femtosecond lenticule extraction (FLEx)*.[2,3] The technique evolved over the years to a novel flap-less procedure called *small incision lenticule extraction (SMILE)*, which rapidly gained popularity with favorable outcomes.[4] The VisuMax femtosecond laser system (Carl Zeiss Meditec, Jena, Germany) is the only laser platform approved for the creation of an intrastromal refractive lenticule.[5] A complete and thorough knowledge of the machine and its parameters is of paramount importance before undertaking any refractive surgery. This chapter is aimed at describing in detail the machine, its components and the pretreatment settings which are required for successful completion of the procedure.

BASIC PRINCIPLE OF THE MACHINE

Femtosecond lasers are near-infrared lasers with ultrashort duration of pulses to the order of 10^{-15} seconds which result in minimal collateral tissue damage. They work on the principle of *photodisruption*. Photodisruption involves the nonlinear absorption of laser energy in the target, which results in optical breakdown of the tissue. The highly focused femtosecond laser pulses form plasma of free electrons and ionized molecules at the laser focus and the phenomenon is called *laser-induced optical breakdown (LIOB)*. The rapid expansion of plasma results in the formation of cavitation bubbles, which enlarge and coalesce to allow separation of tissue with minimal damage to the surrounding tissue.

The VisuMax femtosecond laser system (Fig. 4.1) delivers focused pattern of femtosecond pulses on to the cornea and cuts at a precise pre-decided depth and position.

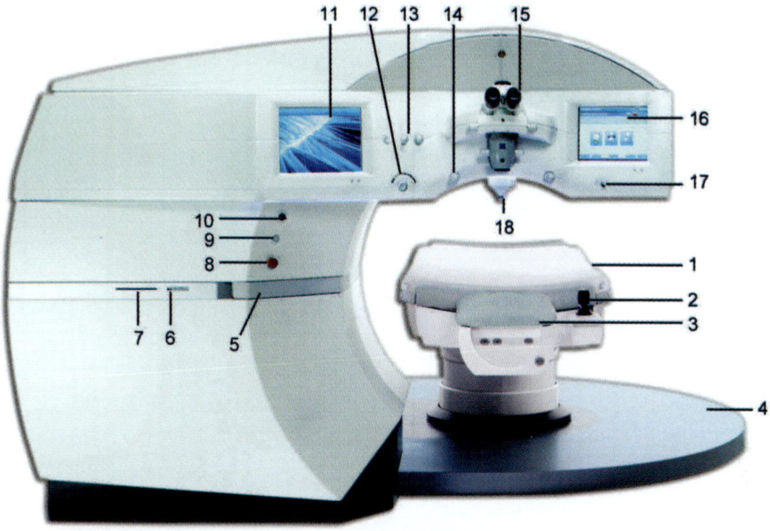

1 Patient supporting system
2 Joystick
3 Headrest
4 Rotating platform
5 Keyboard tray
6 USB 2.0 interface
7 DVD RAM drive
8 Emergency stop button
9 System start button
10 Key switch
11 Monitor (system control)
12 Vacuum suction control and display
13 Illumination control
14 Slit illumination system
15 Surgical microscope with integrated video camera
16 Touch screen (procedure control)
17 Treatment pack vacuum connection
18 Laser aperture

Fig. 4.1: VisuMax femtosecond laser system (Carl Zeiss Meditec, Jena, Germany).

The machine weighs 870 kg and serves as a one-stop station for SMILE unlike femtosecond laser-assisted in situ keratomileusis (FS-LASIK) that requires two separate stations for excimer and femtosecond laser.

UNDERSTANDING THE MACHINE

The functional components of the VisuMax femtosecond laser system are highlighted and summarized in Table 4.1 (Figs. 4.1 and 4.2). The machine is switched on by pushing the system start button, followed by inserting the key in the key switch. The machine houses a computer unit, laser arm and vacuum system, microscope, patient supporting system and a foot switch. Different illumination systems are integrated in the machine, including diffuse, slit and infrared illumination (Fig. 4.3). The treatment pack is a single-use disposable contact lens with attached tubing that provides the interface between the patient and the machine (Fig. 4.4).

Computer Unit

An integrated computer with a graphic user-interface enables easy control of the laser keratome (Fig. 4.3). The graphic user interface allows the user

Table 4.1: Components of VisuMax femtosecond laser system

Component	*Description*
Computer unit	▪ In-built graphic user interface ▪ Feeding treatment data ▪ Two output screens i. *Left screen*: Treatment planning and live monitoring ii. *Right screen*: Graphic user interface, displays progress of treatment.
Laser arm and vacuum system	▪ Directs the laser radiation from the laser unit to the exit aperture ▪ Vacuum system provides attachment for contact lens onto laser aperture, and fixes the eye on the contact lens
Microscope	▪ Surgical microscope ▪ Switches between observation and treatment mode ▪ Diffuse, infrared and slit illumination ▪ In-built video recording
Patient supporting system	▪ Operating table with headrest ▪ *Three positions*: (1) starting, (2) observation and (3) treatment positions ▪ Allows comfortable patient positioning ▪ Movements controlled automatically by laser keratome, manually by joystick
Foot switch	▪ Controls laser delivery • *Press*: Opens laser shutter and activates laser delivery • *Release*: Closes laser shutter and stops laser
Treatment pack	▪ Single-use disposable contact lens with attached tubing ▪ Provides interface between the patient and the machine ▪ Three sizes: (1) small, (2) medium and (3) large (*S*, *M* and *L*), based on white-to-white diameter of the patient.

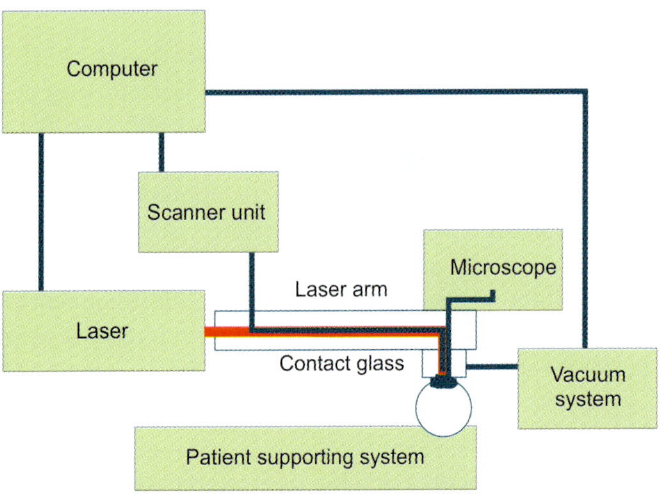

Fig. 4.2: Functional components of the VisuMax femtosecond laser system.

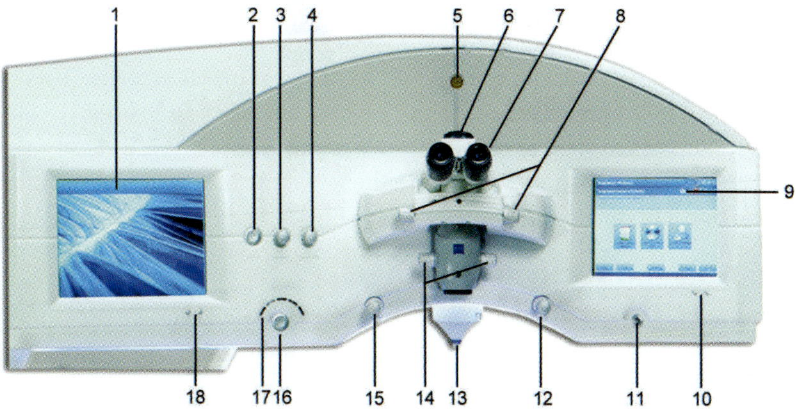

1 Monitor (system control)
2 Infrared illumination
3 Illumination control (observation)
4 Illumination control (treatment)
5 Laser radiation emission indicator
6 Interpupillary distance adjustment
7 Eyepiece
8 Fine focus adjustment
9 Touch screen (procedure control)
10, 18 Brightness control
11 Vacuum suction connection for treatment pack
12, 15 Slit illumination system
13 Laser treatment aperture
14 Magnification control (Objective)
16 Vacuum suction control element (on/off)
17 Vacuum suction display

Fig. 4.3: Control elements and display on the laser keratome.

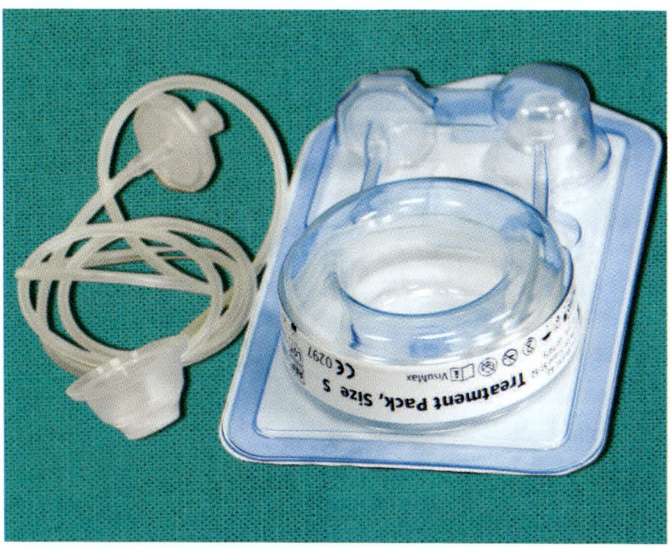

Fig. 4.4: Single-use treatment pack with contact glass interface.

to enter the patient details and preoperative data, as well as saves the treatment data. The laser settings and treatment parameters may be modified by the surgeon as per requirements. Other computers control and monitor the internal sequences.

The VisuMax femtosecond laser system for ReLEx SMILE is user friendly with two computer output screens. Instructions for the surgeon and the real-time status of treatment are displayed on the touch screens. The left screen is for treatment planning and live monitoring of the surgery, while the screen on the right side of the surgeon is the graphic user interface and shows the progress of the treatment. The progress of treatment planning can also be analyzed on this screen graphically.

Laser Arm and Vacuum System

Laser arm directs the laser radiation from the laser unit to the exit aperture of the treatment lens. A contact glass is coupled to the patient's eye connecting it to the laser exit aperture.

The vacuum system provides the attachment for the contact lens onto the laser aperture, and fixes the eye on the contact lens. It stabilizes patient's eye and ensures that the eye is aligned with the contact glass and the laser exit aperture.

Suction is initiated by pressing the top button on the joystick. The vacuum level is monitored by in-built pressure sensors and displayed by the blue LED scale on the vacuum suction pressure display. The presence of four or more blue bars on the LED display denotes an adequate quality of the generated vacuum. Laser application is possible only after generation of adequate vacuum.

Patient Supporting System

The patient supporting system consists of an operating table along with the headrest. It is mobile and the position is controlled automatically by the laser keratome and manually by the joystick. Three positions of the patient supporting system are: (1) the starting position, (2) the observation position and (3) the treatment position. It allows comfortable positioning of the patient and ensures accurate and precise movement during the surgery.

Surgical Microscope

The surgical microscope with a binocular eyepiece aids in ocular examination, preparation for surgery as well as observation and completion of the surgical process. The inter-pupillary distance, magnification (objective: 0.4–2.5×, eyepiece: 10×) and fine-focus can be adjusted with the help of in-built knobs. Integrated video camera in the microscope aids in recording the surgical videos. The provision of an integrated slit-illumination system allows an on-table assessment of the interface at the end of surgery. The surgical microscope can shift between the treatment position (for docking and laser delivery) and observation position (for lenticule dissection and extraction), in concordance with the movement of the patient supporting system.

Foot Switch

The foot switch is connected to the machine and is used to control the laser delivery. Pressing the foot switch opens the laser shutter and activates the laser treatment. Releasing the foot switch closes the laser shutter and stops the laser treatment.

Illumination Systems (Fig. 4.3)

- *Observation position*: The patient's eye is illuminated by the microscope lamp in observation position beneath the surgical microscope. Two knurled knobs are present that allow the adjustment of brightness levels by turning the knobs.
- *Treatment position*: The patient's eye is illuminated by the illumination at the contact glass mount in the treatment position beneath the therapy lens. The brightness can be adjusted by turning the knurled knob, and illumination can be turned on or off by pushing the knob.
- *Slit illumination*: Slit illumination is available on the left or right-hand side of the surgical microscope with a fixed slit dimension (0.5 mm × 12 mm). It is activated by pushing on the knurled knob on either side, which switches off the diffuse white illumination and activates the slit illumination. The slit position and angle can be adjusted by rotating the knurled knob. It is switched off by pushing the knob again.
- *Infrared illumination*: The infrared button can be used to switch between white light and infrared illumination. It aids in centering the contact lens during docking. The infrared image is displayed on the left-hand side monitor.

Treatment Pack

The *treatment pack* (Fig. 4.4) refers to the single use curved treatment interface or contact lens which is docked to the patient's eye and aligns it to the laser exit beam aperture. It consists of a patient interface with a contact glass, connecting tubing, filter and a vacuum connection which is subsequently attached to the control panel.

The curved nature of the interface ensures that the corneal apex does not shift during applanation. It is illuminated at the time of surgery and serves as an illuminated fixation target for patient eye alignment. It is available in three sizes: (1) small, (2) medium and (3) large (*S*, *M* and *L*). The choice of size of treatment pack for surgery depends on the white-to-white diameter of the patient. The diameter of the suction ring should be less than the effective white-to-white diameter of the patient. Moreover, the effective maximum cap diameter possible with the selected treatment pack should be more than or at least equal to the proposed cap diameter. The smallest possible treatment pack should ideally be selected. If the ring is too large, it may cause suction on

Table 4.2: Manufacturer recommended treatment pack size and the minimum white-to-white diameters for small incision lenticule extraction

Size of treatment pack	*Small**	*Medium*	*Large*
Minimum WTW diameter	11.2	11.7	12.4

Note: *Universally preferred size for WTW < 11.2 mm.
(WTW: White-to-white diameter).

adjacent conjunctiva and lead to subconjunctival hemorrhage, conjunctival bogging or premature abortion of the treatment due to loss of suction.

The recommended treatment pack size as per the white-to-white measurement is given in Table 4.2.

Safety Systems

The laser keratome has an outer protective housing to prevent inadvertent laser exposure to the medical personnel. A beam attenuator is installed on the laser keratome as well as the viewing optics to limit the radiation exposure. An internal power supply provides a failsafe mechanism in the event of intraoperative power failures, and can provide an uninterrupted power supply for up to 3 minutes.

An emergency stop button provides the option to immediately abort the procedure if required. A key switch switches on the laser keratome and boots up the computer on inserting the key. It requires the insertion of a key during the surgical procedure, and laser cannot be triggered after removing the key. The laser radiation warning indicator is illuminated when the laser is being fired.

UNDERSTANDING THE LASER PARAMETERS

The VisuMax laser system has in-built surgical applications for FLEx, flap, circle, keratoplasty and intracorneal ring segment incisions along with that of ReLEx SMILE. Hence, the first step in planning is to choose the right procedure. This chapter deals with planning of the ReLEx SMILE procedure.

Treatment planning involves accurate entry of the treatment data which includes the lenticule and the cap parameters (Figs. 4.5 and 4.6). Lenticule dimensions mainly depend on the manifest refraction, optical zone (OZ) diameter, transition zone (TZ) and minimum lenticule thickness predefined. All these parameters need to be entered while planning the treatment. The lenticule and cap treatment parameters are summarized in Table 4.3.

Lenticule Parameters (Table 4.3 and Fig. 4.5)

- *Optical zone* diameter ranges from 5 mm to 8 mm. The OZ is selected on the basis of pupil size, and may be increased in patients with a large

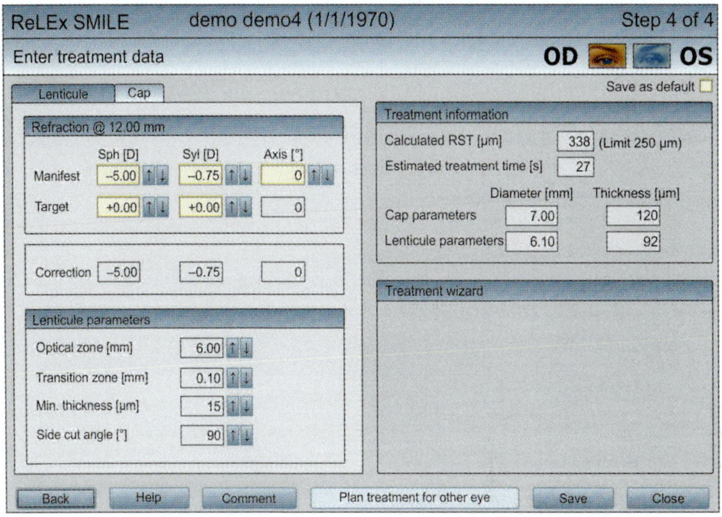

Fig. 4.5: Lenticule parameters for small incision lenticule extraction.

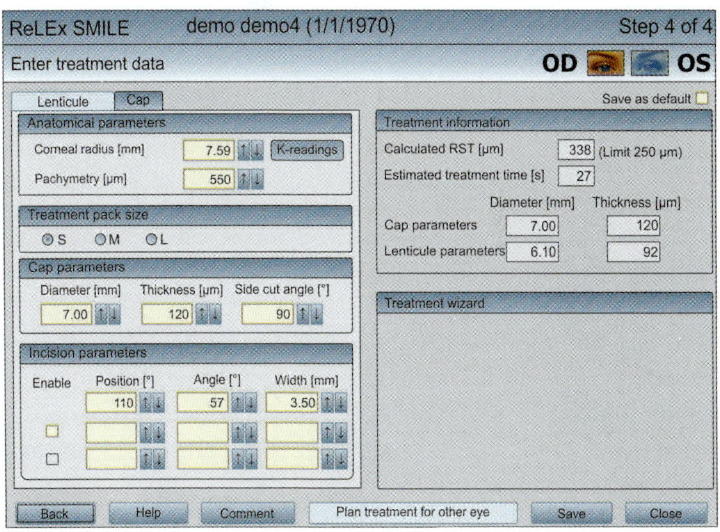

Fig. 4.6: Cap parameters for small incision lenticule extraction.

mesopic pupil. It is usually set at 6–6.5 mm for average corneal diameters of 10–12 mm.

- *Transition zone* is preset and depends on the manifest refraction. In case of purely spherical errors, the machine automatically sets the value at 0 while in case of any cylinder, the value changes to 0.10 mm.
- *Lenticule diameter* is the sum of OZ diameter and the TZ.

$$\text{Lenticule diameter} = \text{OZ} + \text{TZ}.$$

Table 4.3: Treatment parameters for small incision lenticule extraction using VisuMax femtosecond laser system

Parameter	***Range***
Cap parameters	
▪ Cap thickness	100–160 μm
▪ Cap diameter	6–9.6 mm
▪ Incision position	0–359°
▪ Incision width	2–5 mm
▪ Cap side-cut angle	45–135°
Lenticule parameters	
▪ Lenticule diameter	5–8 mm
▪ Transition zone	0.10 mm for CYL 0 for SPH
▪ Minimum lenticule thickness	10–30 μm
▪ Lenticule side cut angle	90–179°

- *Minimum thickness of the lenticule (LT_{min})* in myopic SMILE refers to the peripheral edge of the lenticule. While the central thickness varies with the refractive error, the peripheral minimum thickness can be prefixed. It can be altered by the user as per surgeon's ease in handling thinner lenticule and in cases of lower refractive errors. In most cases, the minimum thickness of lenticule is fixed at 15 μm, though it can be increased to 25-30 μm in case of lower refractive errors where a thinner lenticule is expected. The height of lenticule side cut is equal to the lenticule minimum thickness.
- *Total lenticule thickness (LT_{total})* is the sum of minimum thickness of lenticule (LT_{min}) and the amount of tissue (n) that will be removed as per the amount of refractive error. This is usually extrapolated from Munnerlyn formula and is considered to be around 13 μm for every diopter correction at 6 mm OZ.

$$LT_{total} = LT_{min} + n.$$

Cap Parameters

Cap parameters that need to be entered in the graphic-user interface during treatment planning include the keratometry and the thinnest corneal thickness measured (Table 4.3 and Fig. 4.6).

- *Cap diameter* is 0.5-1 mm oversized from the OZ diameter. The effective maximum cap diameter ranges from 6 mm to 9.6 mm, and depends on the size of treatment pack, cap thickness, radius of the corneal curvature and the side cut angle.

- *Cap thickness* is 120 microns in standard cases, though it may be varied from 100 microns to 160 microns depending upon the refractive error and corneal thickness.
- *Cap side-cut* is usually placed between 90° and 180° depending on surgeon's dexterity and ease of functioning. The incision width may vary from 2 mm to 5 mm, with wider incision for initial cases. One or two cap side-cut incisions may be selected, depending upon the surgeon preference.
- *Residual stromal bed thickness (RSBT)* is calculated by the machine using in-built nomograms for lenticule thickness according to refractive error. The acceptable limit for RSBT is 250–280 microns.
- *Keratometry* is entered as per the corneal topography of the patient. Both the radius of curvature and the dioptric power may be entered.

Selection of Laser Settings

Laser settings are preset in the machine and depend on the mode selected (Table 4.4). Three modes of treatment are available, that is (1) *Standard,* (2) *Fast* and (3) *Expert modes.* The *standard mode* refers to the default laser parameters set by the manufacturers. The *fast mode* may be altered only by the application specialists, and consists of pre-set laser parameters customized according to the region. The *expert mode* has modifiable laser settings which may be optimized by the surgeon, according to the surgeon preference and patient response. The expert mode allows the surgeon to make modifications in the laser parameters of the fast mode (which have been set by the application specialist for that region), within a certain range. It is advisable to consult the application specialist regarding the optimal laser and energy settings.

- *Spot spacing*
  Spot spacing refers to the distance between two adjacent laser spots (Fig. 4.7) and ranges from 2.0 μm to 4.5 μm. In the expert mode, the surgeon may modify spot spacing in steps of ±0.1 microns each, by a maximum of ±0.5 microns.
- *Track spacing*
  Track spacing refers to the distance between two laser spots in adjacent tracks (Fig. 4.7) and ranges from 2.0 μm to 4.5 μm. In the expert mode, the surgeon may modify track spacing in steps of ±0.1 microns each, by a maximum of ±0.5 microns.
- *Pulse energy*
  Pulse energy defines the size of the cavitation bubbles which are produced during femtosecond laser cuts. It lies in the range of 100–260 nJ (recommended 100–160 nJ). Energy offset is set for each cut separately in expert mode.

  1 Energy offset = 5 nJ pulse energy.

Table 4.4: Laser parameters used for small incision lenticule extraction

Parameter	**Range**	**Expert mode[1]**	**Standard mode[2]**	**Fast mode[3]**
Pulse energy	100–260 nJ (recommended 100–160 nJ)	140–200 nJ	130 nJ	170 nJ
Energy offset (1 offset = 5 nJ)	20–52	28–40	26	34
Track distance	2.0–4.5 µm	▪ Lenticule and cap cuts: 4.5 ± 0.5 µm ▪ Lenticule and cap side-cuts: 2 ± 0.5 µm	▪ 3 µm for lenticule and cap cuts ▪ 2 µm for lenticule and cap side-cuts	▪ 4.5 µm for lenticule and cap cuts ▪ 2 µm for lenticule and cap side-cuts
Spot distance	2.0–4.5 µm	▪ Lenticule and cap cuts: 4.5 ± 0.5 µm ▪ Lenticule and cap side-cuts: 2 ± 0.5 µm	▪ 3 µm for lenticule and cap cuts ▪ 2 µm for lenticule and cap side-cuts	▪ 4.5 µm for lenticule and cap cuts ▪ 2 µm for lenticule and cap side-cuts
Scan direction	Spiral in for lenticule cut; spiral out for cap cut	Fixed	Fixed	Fixed
Scan mode	Single	Fixed	Fixed	Fixed
Wavelength	1,043 nm	Fixed	Fixed	Fixed
Pulse duration	220–580 fs	Fixed	Fixed	Fixed
Laser repetition rate	500 kHz	Fixed	Fixed	Fixed

[1] The expert mode allows the surgeon to vary the “fast” mode settings within a certain range.
[2] The standard settings are preset by the manufacturer.
[3] The fast settings are set by the application specialist, and may vary from surgeon to surgeon.

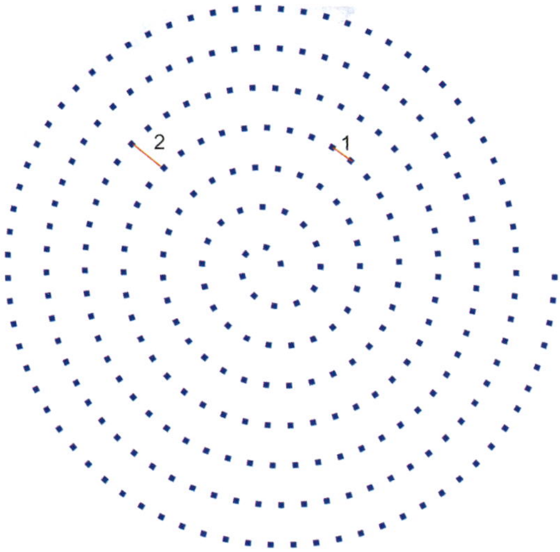

Fig. 4.7: Concentric arrangement of laser spots depicting spot distance (1) and track distance (2).

The energy offset may lie in the range of 20–52 (recommended 20–32), and may be titrated by the surgeon as per the observed clinical effects, in terms of smooth dissection and minimal opaque bubble layer (OBL) formation. The expert mode allows the surgeon to modify energy offset by ±6 steps (total energy ± 30 nJ).

- *Scan direction and mode*

  Scan direction refers to the direction of the spiral that the laser follows while making the cuts. Conventionally, it is spiral in for posterior plane and spiral out for anterior plane. In SMILE, for the lenticule formation, these spirals must be elliptical and not circular.

  Scan mode is preset as "single", and refers to the creation of the entire lenticule in one go. Scan mode can be changed only by the application specialist, and may be single or double; however, only single scan mode is preferred.

These settings affect the amount of energy being delivered to the cornea and the quality of cut as well as duration of surgery (Table 4.5). Decreased laser *spot distance or track distance* will deliver the laser spots close to each other and hence, cumulatively more energy is delivered to cornea. This may produce smoother cuts with more complete dissection and possibly less adhesions. On the other hand, widely spaced spots or tracks may lead to more intraoperative difficulty owing to increased possibility of adhesions. Higher *pulse energy* for cuts has been seen to be associated with suboptimal visual recovery and increased higher order aberrations. OBL is seen to occur with both excessively high energy and low energy. In case of higher pulse energy,

Table 4.5: Effect of spot distance, track distance and pulse energy on small incision lenticule extraction

Parameter	*Effect*
Decreased spot distance, track distance	▪ More energy delivered to cornea ▪ Smoother cuts ▪ More complete dissection, less adhesions
Increased spot distance, track distance	▪ Less energy delivered to cornea ▪ Less smooth cuts ▪ May have more adhesions
Decreased pulse energy	▪ Less energy delivered to cornea ▪ Less smooth cuts ▪ May have more adhesions ▪ May have faster visual recovery ▪ Better quality of postoperative vision
Increased pulse energy	▪ More energy delivered to cornea ▪ Smoother cuts ▪ More complete dissection, less adhesions ▪ Increased risk of dense opaque bubble layer ▪ May have prolonged visual recovery ▪ May affect postoperative quality of vision

large cavitation bubbles and shock waves spread the corneal collagen lamellae apart with force and lead to OBL formation which shoots ahead of the laser beam. OBL may also occur when the pulse energy is much below the accepted limit though such OBLs are less dense and patchy and appear late during laser delivery.

MAINTENANCE OF THE MACHINE AND SET-UP CONDITIONS

Refractive surgery modules such as VisuMax femtosecond laser system require accurate temperature and humidity conditions for smooth functioning (Table 4.6). Maintenance and regular servicing are of utmost importance. The well being of the machine in several ways decides the surgical outcomes as well. Hence, only trained personnel should perform the calibration, maintenance and service of the machine.

VisuMax femtosecond laser system is a 870 kg refractive surgery module that should ideally be placed in a room with adequate floor area. The permitted range of ambient temperature lies between 18°C and 25°C and humidity in the range of 30–70%. A 100–240 V electrical connection is required for the functioning of the machine. It should be placed away from inflammable products. Cell phones should be kept away from the laser operation theatre (OT) as their signals may interfere with laser delivery. Sterilization and disinfection of OT is important and standard OT practices must be followed for the same.

Table 4.6: Technical specifications of VisuMax femtosecond laser system for performing small incision lenticule extraction	
Specifications	***Value***
Weight	870 kg
Electrical connection	100–240 V
Room temperature	18–25°C
Ambient humidity	30–70%
Other accessories	▪ Single use treatment packs ▪ Keratoplasty adapter (for wet lab training and performing femtosecond keratoplasty)

An internal calibration is automatically performed by the system (system test) prior to the surgical procedure, in order to ensure the highest accuracy of the cut surface geometry.

CONCLUSION

Understanding the machine and its settings lays out the first step toward mastering any surgery. SMILE is a novel entry in the world of refractive surgery; hence, not many surgeons are yet acquainted with the machine. Complete knowledge of the principle and various components of the machine as well as the laser and surgical parameters can simplify the procedure for the surgeons, especially the beginners.

REFERENCES

1. Sekundo W, Kunert K, Russmann C, et al. First efficacy and safety study of femtosecond lenticule extraction for the correction of myopia. J Cataract Refract Surg. 2008;34:1513-20.
2. Reinstein DZ, Archer TJ, Gobbe M, et al. Accuracy and reproducibility of Artemis central flap thickness and visual outcomes of LASIK with the Carl Zeiss Meditec VisuMax femtosecond laser and MEL 80 excimer laser platforms. J Refract Surg. 2010;26:107-19.
3. Vestergaard A, Ivarsen A, Asp S, et al. Femtosecond (FS) laser vision correction procedure for moderate to high myopia: a prospective study of ReLEx® flex and comparison with a retrospective study of FS-laser in situ keratomileusis. Acta Ophthalmol. 2013;91:355-62.
4. Sekundo W, Kunert KS, Blum M. Small incision corneal refractive surgery using the small incision lenticule extraction (SMILE) procedure for the correction of myopia and myopic astigmatism: results of a 6 month prospective study. Br J Ophthalmol. 2011;95:335-9.
5. VisuMax Femtosecond Laser. Small Incision Lenticule Extraction (SMILE) procedure for the correction of myopia: professional use information. [online] Available at: https://www.accessdata.fda.gov/cdrh_docs/pdf15/P150040D.pdf [Accessed July 2017].

Chapter 5

Surgical Technique of Small Incision Lenticule Extraction

Manpreet Kaur, Jeewan S Titiyal

INTRODUCTION

Small incision lenticule extraction (SMILE) employs femtosecond laser to create an intrastromal refractive lenticule which is then dissected from the stromal bed and extracted through a small side cut incision of 2–5 mm width. The surgical technique is more challenging than flap-based corneal ablative procedures and associated with a steep learning curve. In this chapter, we have comprehensively described the conventional surgical technique of SMILE along with the preoperative patient preparation and postoperative regimen. The modifications of surgical techniques to facilitate easy lenticule extraction have also been discussed. Specialized instruments developed for lenticule separation and extraction have been described.

PREOPERATIVE CONSIDERATIONS

The preoperative considerations and patient preparation are outlined in Table 5.1.

Patient Selection and Evaluation

The factors pertaining to case selection for SMILE have been detailed in Chapter 2 "Patient Counseling and Preoperative Evaluation". A thorough preoperative workup should include both cycloplegic and manifest refraction. The white-to-white diameter should be ascertained to determine the size of the contact lens. Topography should be done to screen the presence of forme fruste keratoconus and the cases at high risk for postoperative ectasia. A detailed anterior segment and fundus examination is essential to rule out any ocular comorbidity or posterior segment pathology.

Patient Counseling and Informed Consent

A thorough preoperative counseling is essential to determine the patient expectations from the procedure and inform them about the potential pros and cons. Unrealistic expectations need to be addressed. A written informed

Table 5.1: Preoperative preparation in a case of small incision lenticule extraction

Preoperative considerations	*Steps*
Patient selection—comprehensive workup	▪ Refraction—manifest and cycloplegic ▪ White-to-white diameter ▪ Topography (Orbscan/Pentacam) ▪ Anterior segment evaluation-slit lamp/intraocular pressure ▪ Fundus—periphery screening
Patient counseling and consent	▪ Written informed consent ▪ Explain pros and cons ▪ Address unrealistic patient expectations ▪ Explain procedure—what patient is expected to do during surgery
Preoperative medications	▪ Topical antibiotic (moxifloxacin 0.5% one drop) ▪ Topical anesthesia (proparacaine 0.5% one drop—three times at 5-minute intervals, 15 minutes before surgery)
Patient positioning	▪ Supine—arms on side/gently folded over abdomen ▪ Straight ahead gaze ▪ Iris plane parallel to ground ▪ Gently tilt face or chin if prominent nasal bridge
Clean and drape	▪ Periocular skin and lids—10% povidone-iodine ▪ Conjunctival fornix—5% povidone-iodine ▪ Sterile disposable drape ▪ Wire speculum or aspirating speculum to separate eyelids

consent is necessary. It would be wise to remember the maxim "*not written is not done*", and ensure a detailed documentation of the consent as well as the entire surgical procedure to prevent any future medicolegal complications. The patient should be explained the entire surgical procedure, as well as what the patient is expected to do during surgery. The patient has to fixate on the green fixation light, avoid sudden, jerky ocular movements and not squeeze the eyelids during surgery. A well-informed patient is more likely to cooperate during surgery and lead to a smooth, uneventful completion of the procedure.

Preoperative Preparation

We prefer to instill a drop of topical antibiotic (moxifloxacin 0.5%) in both eyes in the preoperative period. Topical proparacaine 0.5% is instilled in both eyes to provide anesthesia. One drop is instilled in both eyes at 5 minute intervals for a total of three times, beginning from 15 minutes before surgery. Excessive instillation of topical anesthesia should be avoided as it causes loosening of the corneal epithelium, and may predispose to epithelial defects and formation of black spots.

Patient Positioning and Draping

The operating table is shifted perpendicular to the machine to allow the patient to lie on it (Fig. 5.1A). The patient is asked to lie supine on the operating table, with both arms either positioned straight at the sides, or gently folded to lie over the abdomen. The operating table is then aligned with the laser keratome with the head-rest below the laser firing arm during surgery (Fig. 5.1B).

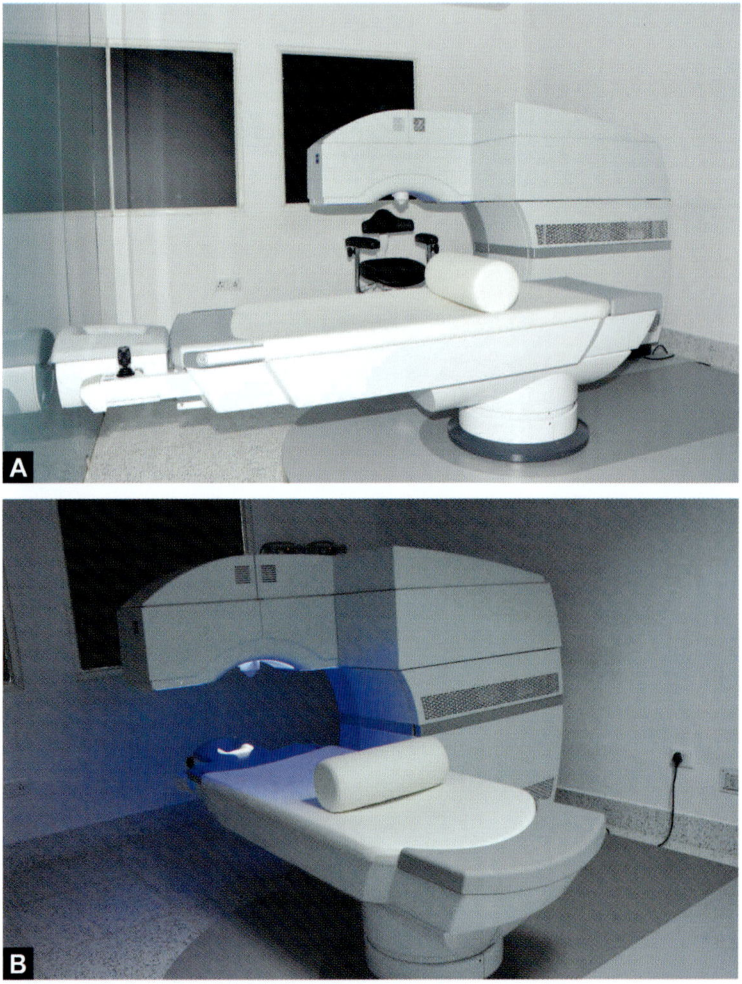

Figs. 5.1A and B: Position of the patient supporting system. (A) The operating table is shifted perpendicular to the machine to allow the patient to lie supine on the table; and (B) The operating table is aligned with the laser keratome with the head-rest below the laser firing arm during surgery.

The patient's head is positioned so that the iris plane of both eyes is parallel to the ground. In cases with a prominent nasal bridge, the chin and face position may be gently tilted so as to ensure that the nose does not interfere with docking.

We prefer to operate both eyes sequentially. The right eye is operated first as per convention, followed by the left. Some surgeons prefer to complete femtosecond laser application in both eyes first, followed by lenticule extraction in both eyes. However, the reference bubble layer may disappear in the waiting period and this may create difficulties in identification of the dissection planes. We prefer to extract the lenticule immediately after the femtosecond laser application.

The periocular skin and eyelids are cleaned with 10% povidone-iodine. One drop of 5% povidone-iodine solution is instilled in the conjunctival fornix. The periocular surface is allowed to dry, and a sterile disposable drape is applied to the eye being operated first. A universal wire-speculum is inserted to separate the eyelids and ensure adequate exposure of the operating field. A wire speculum has the advantage of being light-weight and does not exert undue pressure on the globe. An aspirating speculum may be used to ensure continuous drainage of excessive fluid. A solid-blade speculum may be useful in cases with loose conjunctival tissue to mechanically hold the conjunctiva away from the central field.

SURGICAL TECHNIQUE

The surgical procedure involves docking, femtosecond laser application followed by lenticule dissection and extraction (Table 5.2 and 1 to 10 and 20).

Table 5.2: Stepwise surgical technique of small incision lenticule extraction

Surgical steps	***Procedure***
Docking (1 and 2)	▪ Contact lens (S/M/L) as per patient's WTW diameter ▪ Patient fixates on green internal fixation light ▪ Contact lens acurvates ocular surface ▪ Suction initiated
Femtosecond laser application (1 and 20)	500 kHz femtosecond laser ▪ *Lenticule cut*: Outside-in pattern, diameter 6–7 mm ▪ *Lenticule side-cut*: Minimum thickness 10–30 microns ▪ *Cap cut*: 0.5–1 mm larger than lenticule cut, inside-out pattern ▪ *Cap side-cut*: 2–5 mm width, 110°, 1–2 in number
Lenticule dissection and extraction (1 to 10 and 20)	▪ Side-cut opened with hooked end of dissector ▪ *Lenticule edge identified*: Upper and lower edges delineated with hooked end of dissector ▪ Anterior lenticule plane separated with blunt dissector ▪ Posterior lenticule plane separated with blunt dissector ▪ Lenticule extracted through side-cut with microforceps ▪ Pocket irrigated with BSS

(WTW: White-to-white; BSS: Balanced salt solution).

Docking

The contact lens (patient interface) is selected as per the patient's white-to-white diameter (2). Three sizes of contact lenses are available, namely S, M and L. We use "S" size in all our cases due to the smaller white-to-white diameter of Indian eyes (Fig. 5.2A). A mismatch between patient's eye and the contact lens size may predispose to suction loss. The contact glass is attached to a small tube, which is connected to the suction ports on the contact glass at one end and a Luer-Lock connector on the other. The connector is attached to the suction port on the laser keratome.

The eye to be operated is positioned directly beneath the VisuMax femtosecond laser delivery system, and the patient is asked to fixate on the

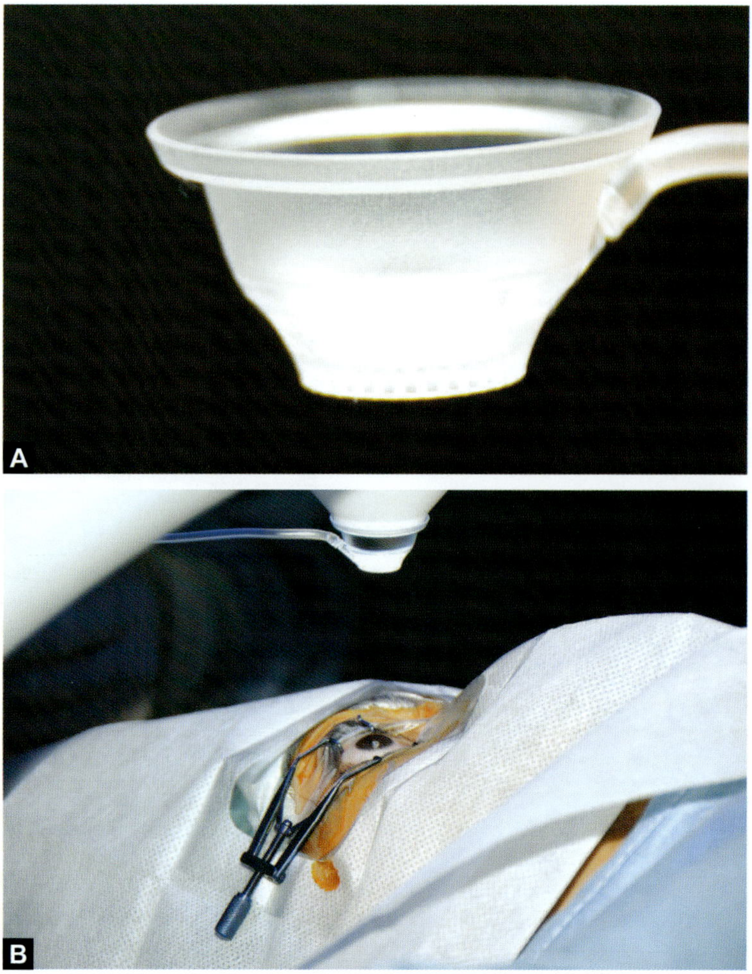

Figs. 5.2A and B: (A) Contact lens and (B) Patient bed is moved up during docking so that the contact lens *"acurvates"* the corneal surface.

green internal fixation light. The patient should be explained that the light will be obscured during femtosecond laser delivery and the patient should not move the eyes to search for the light. The patient bed is moved up during docking so that the contact lens "*acurvates*" the corneal surface (Fig. 5.2B). When the contact lens touches the cornea, a meniscus tear film appears. At this point, the fixation light is clearly visible as the vergence of the fixation beam is focused according to the patient's refraction. The patient is instructed to look directly in the green light, the centering is checked and suction is activated (Fig. 5.3A). In SMILE, the treatment is centered on the coaxially sighted corneal light reflex (CSCLR), which is the reflection of the blinking green light on the cornea. This method allows the patient to auto-centrate the visual axis as well as the corneal vertex to the vertex of the contact glass. The refractive lenticule thus created will be centered on the corneal vertex.

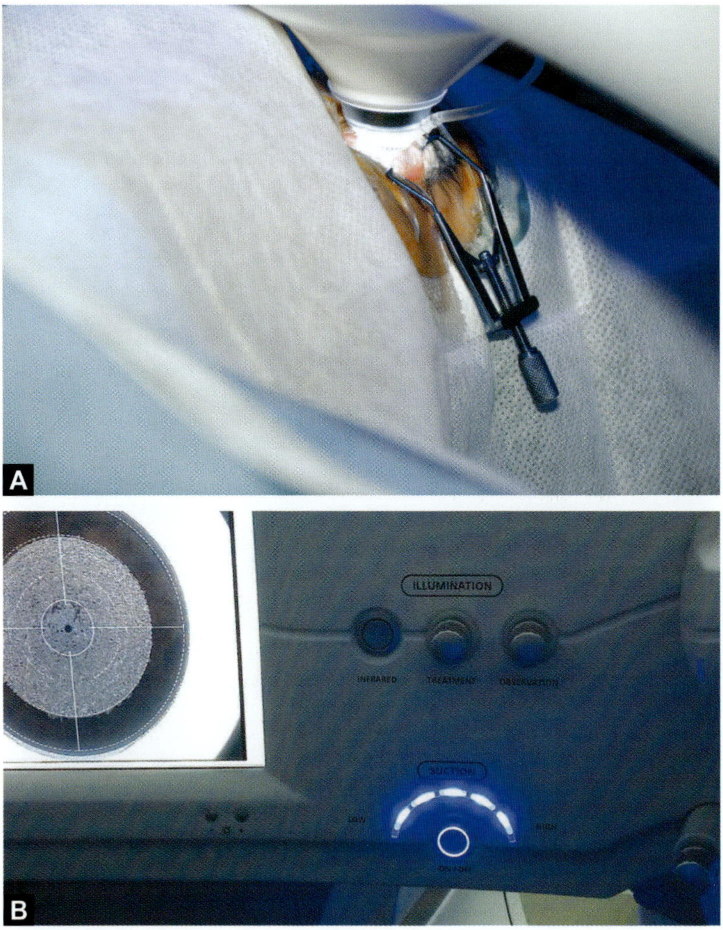

Figs. 5.3A and B: (A) Suction is initiated when the contact lens touches the cornea; and (B) The blue bars on the LED display provide the level of suction generated.

The surgeon should use infrared light to confirm the centration after docking (Figs. 5.4A and B). The relative positions of the corneal reflex and pupil center can be compared to the placido eye image obtained by the Atlas topography scan (Carl Zeiss Meditec, Jena, Germany) to confirm centration. Redocking may be needed in cases with eccentric centration.

A suction pressure of approximately 35 mm Hg is generated to hold the cornea against the contact glass interface (Fig. 5.3B). It raises the intraocular pressure to only 30–80 mm Hg, which allows the intraocular circulation as

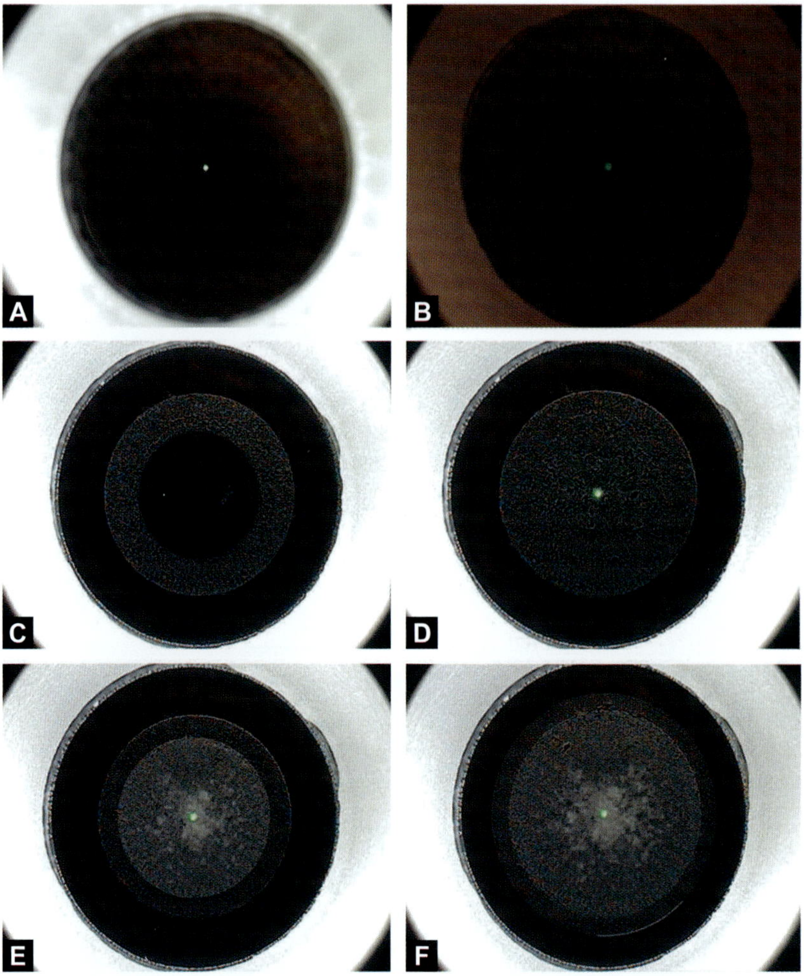

Figs. 5.4A to F: Docking and femtosecond laser delivery in a case of small incision lenticule extraction. (A) Tear meniscus is observed when the contact glass touches the corneal surface, with clear green fixation light; (B) Infrared light is employed to confirm accurate centration of the contact lens with respect to the pupil center and the patient's visual axis; (C) Lenticule cut is created in a spiral-in pattern; (D) Lenticule side-cut is created; (E) Cap cut is created in a spiral-out pattern; and (F) Cap side-cut is created.

well as the patient's vision to be maintained during the procedure.[1,2] The surgeon looks through the surgical microscope during femtosecond laser-assisted lenticule creation, lenticule dissection and extraction.

Femtosecond Laser Application

A 500 kHz femtosecond laser is used to create the refractive lenticule. The laser parameters have been discussed in detail in Chapter 4 (Figs. 5.5A to C). The authors set the femtosecond laser treatment parameters for SMILE at an

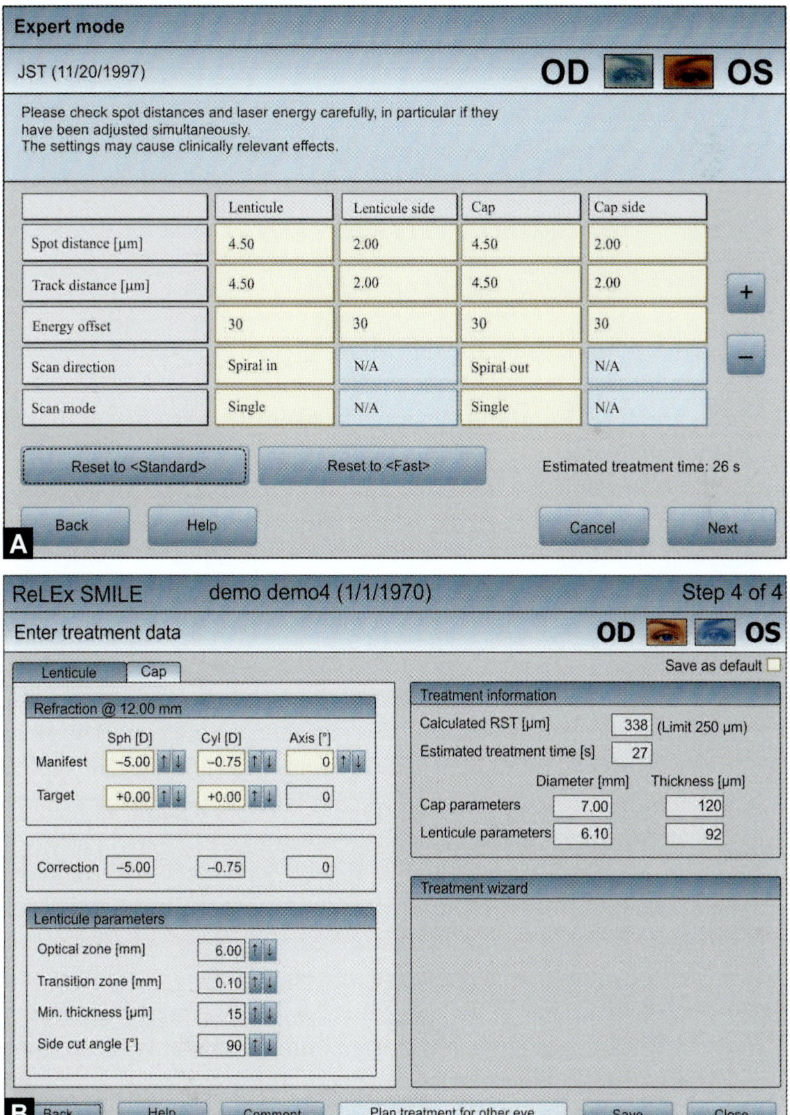

Figs. 5.5A and B: Femtosecond laser settings and treatment parameters. (A) Laser settings in expert mode; (B) Lenticule parameters.

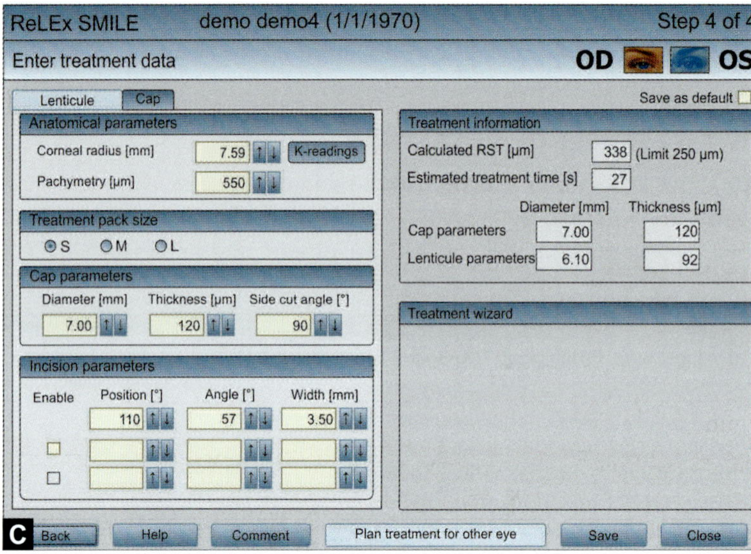

Fig. 5.5C: (C) Cap parameters.

anterior cap depth of 120 µm. The side cut width is set at 4–5 mm for beginners and 2–3 mm for experienced surgeons. The minimum lenticule thickness at the edge is preset at 15 µm, and increased to 20 µm in all cases with spherical equivalent less than 3.0 D. A 6.0 mm optical zone (lenticule cut) is selected with no transition zone for spherical errors and 0.10 mm transition zone for astigmatism. The cap cut is set at 7 mm (1 mm more than the lenticule cut) and the total energy is set at 145–175 nJ. The diameter of the lenticule and cap cut may be altered as per the mesopic pupil size and the white-to-white diameter of the patient.

Four cleavage planes are created as explained below (Figs. 5.4C to F).[3,4]

- *Lenticule cut:* The posterior surface of the lenticule, also known as the lenticule cut, is created first from the periphery to the center by an outside-in (centripetal) pattern of laser delivery. The lenticule cut is the first step as it is the most posterior and will not impede laser delivery or cause light scattering during the creation of more anterior cleavage planes.
- *Lenticule side-cut:* A circumferential vertical incision is made all around the posterior lenticule cut with a depth equivalent to the thickness of the lenticule edge.
- *Cap cut:* The anterior surface of the refractive lenticule is known as the cap cut. The diameter of the cap cut is 0.5–1 mm larger than the lenticule cut. The anterior surface is created from the center to the periphery by an "inside-out" pattern of laser delivery. The laser firing pattern influences the visual recovery rate. An outside-in pattern of lenticule cut with inside-out pattern of cap cut induces minimum microdistortions on

the anterior lenticule surface and promotes early visual recovery when compared to other laser patterns.[5,6]

- *Cap side-cut:* The anterior side-cut or cap side-cut is the last step, and it provides a passage for entry of instruments and lenticule extraction. It has a circumferential length of 2–5 mm with an angle of 110°. One to two side-cut incisions may be selected, and the length adjusted as per the surgeon preference and experience. The location of the side-cut incision is superior in most cases.

The total duration of femtosecond laser delivery is 30–35 seconds (25–28 seconds after a software update) and is not influenced by the magnitude of refractive error. This is due to the fact that the cuts are the same irrespective of the refractive error; they are simply placed further apart for higher magnitude of correction.

At the end of this step, suction is automatically switched off. The contact lens is removed and the patient's eye is moved under the microscope for lenticule extraction.

Lenticule Dissection and Extraction

The side-cut incision is opened with the hooked end of dissector (Fig. 5.6A and 3). Identifying the lenticule edge is the most critical step, and the upper and lower edges of the lenticule are delineated after opening the side-cut, so that the tissue planes are well defined (4 and Figs. 5.6B to D).

The anterior surface of the lenticule is separated first from the overlying cap, followed by posterior lenticule dissection from the stromal bed (Figs. 5.6E to G and 5). After extracting the lenticule, it should be examined for its completeness to rule out any retained peripheral fragments (Figs. 5.6H and I and 6 and 7). The interface may be irrigated with balanced salt solution (Fig. 5.6J). The redundant portions of the cap are distributed evenly to the periphery using a dry Merocel sponge or a blunt instrument (Fig. 5.6K). This step helps to prevent cap microfolds and striae, which may otherwise result from a mismatch between the cap and the stromal bed after lenticule extraction. Either the in-built slit-illumination of the VisuMax laser platform or a standard slit-lamp may be utilized to evaluate the cap apposition at the end of surgery (Fig. 5.6L).

Modified Techniques for Lenticule Dissection and Extraction

Clinical signs have been described that aid in the intraoperative identification of the correct dissection plane, including the "*white ring*" sign and the "*shimmer*" sign (Table 5.3).[7,8]

We prefer a modified technique for identification of the lenticule edge and correct dissection plane. The disparity between the diameter of cap cut and lenticule cut is visible as peripheral rings after femtosecond laser application. After opening the side cut, the anterior and posterior planes are

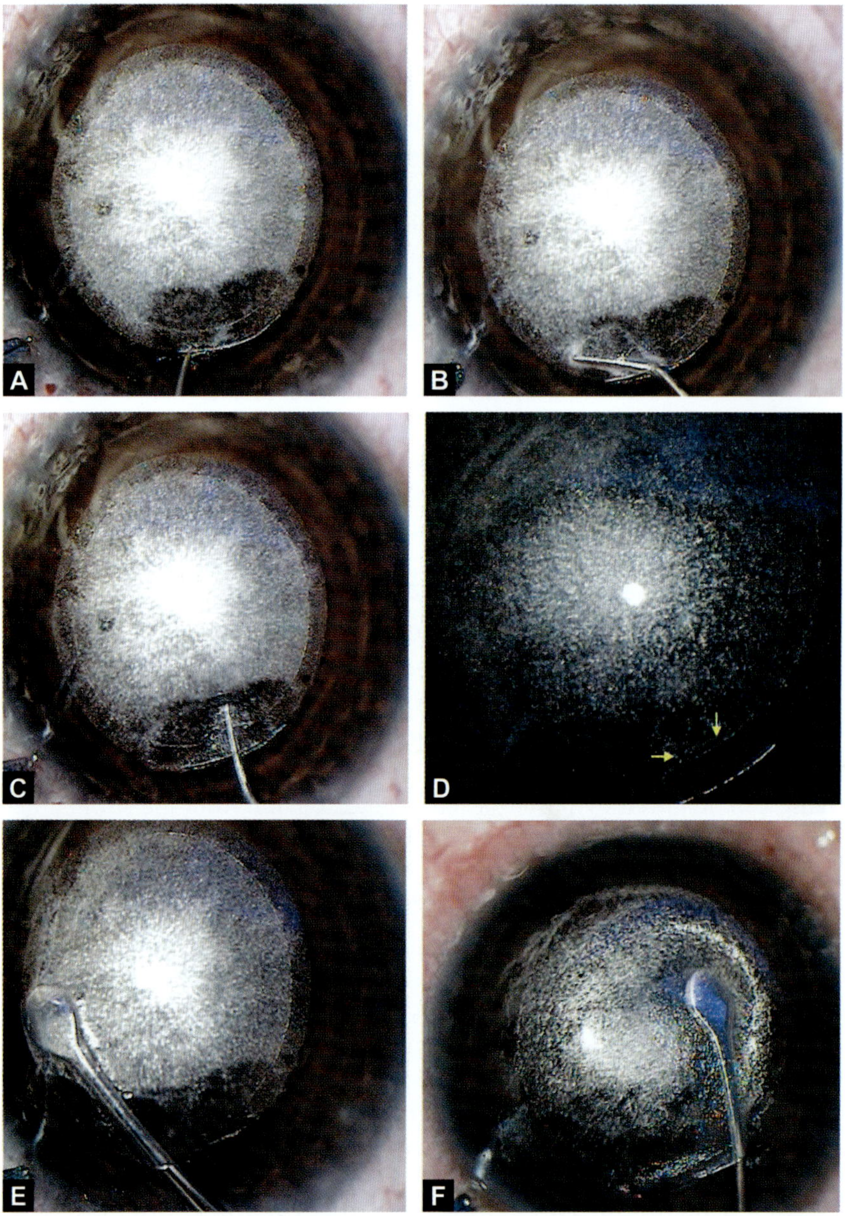

Figs. 5.6A to F: Lenticule dissection and extraction in a case of small incision lenticule extraction. (A) The cap side-cut is opened with the hooked end of a lamellar dissector; (B) The anterior dissection plane is delineated on the left side (for a right-handed surgeon) of the side-cut by inserting the hooked end of lamellar dissector to create a small anterior pocket; (C) The posterior dissection plane is delineated on the right side (for a right-handed surgeon) of the side-cut by inserting the hooked end of lamellar dissector to create a small posterior pocket; (D) Lenticule edge is identified (arrows: lenticule edge); (E and F) The anterior plane is dissected by broad smooth movements of the lamellar dissector, from outside-in.

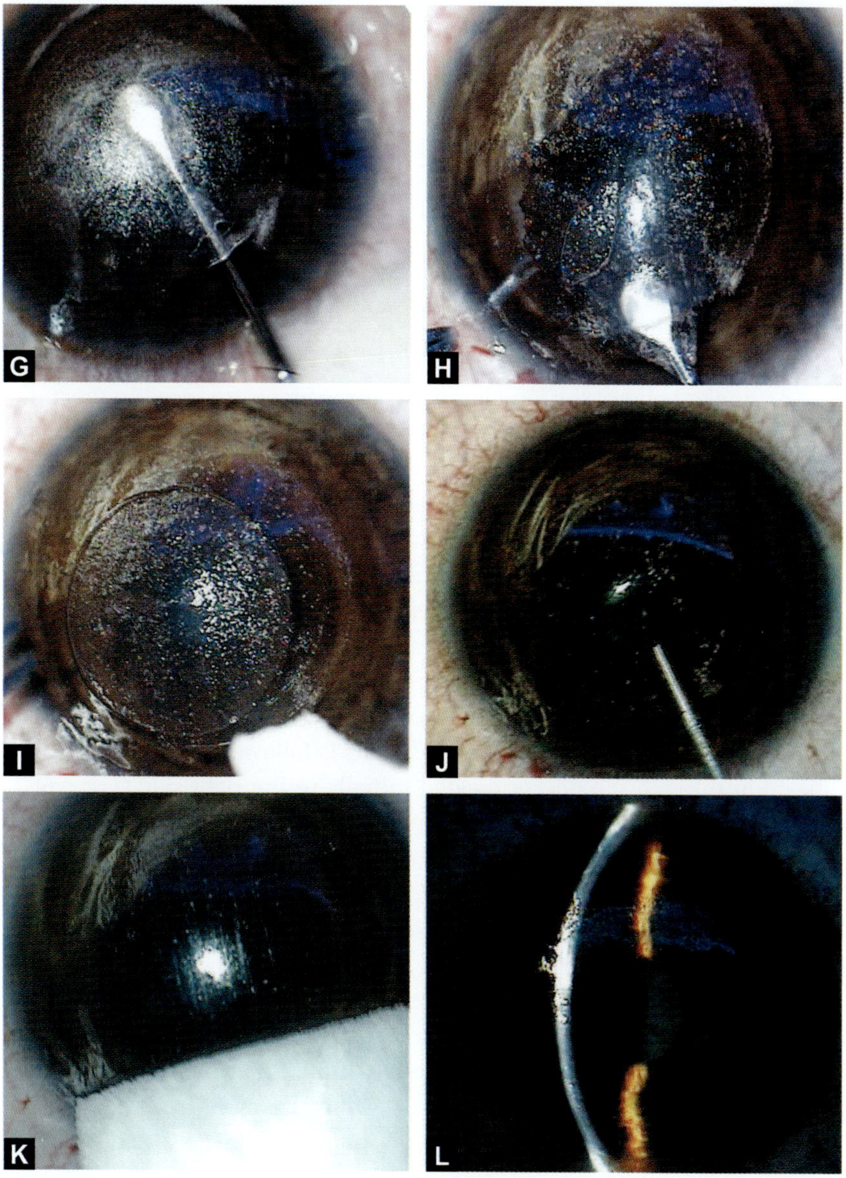

Figs. 5.6G to L: (G) The posterior plane is dissected by the lamellar dissector. Few peripheral undissected areas are left till the end, to provide counter-traction and support during lenticule dissection; (H) Lenticule is extracted through the cap side-cut with the dissector; (I) Lenticule is examined for its completeness; (J) Interface is irrigated with balanced salt solution; (K) Merocel sponge is used to uniformly spread the remaining cap; and (L) In-built slit-illumination is used to assess the apposition at the end of surgery.

delineated in two different directions (Figs. 5.6A to C). A hooked dissector is used to open the cap side-cut incision.

Table 5.3: Clinical signs to identify the dissection plane in small incision lenticule extraction

Clinical signs	*Definition*	*Clinical significance*
White-ring sign	Light reflex from the lenticule side-cut	Identification of the dissection plane-instrument above this ring indicates anterior plane dissection, instrument beneath the white ring indicates posterior plane dissection
Shimmer sign	A bright light reflex around the dissector	Identification of the dissection plane-shimmer sign is only observed when the posterior plane is dissected first, indicating wrong plane of dissection

The hooked end of the lamellar dissector is first introduced in the anterior plane toward the left side (for a right-handed surgeon), ensuring that the dissector reaches the outer margin of the peripheral ring. This step ensures that the dissector is in the anterior plane, and a small circumferential strip is dissected (Fig. 5.6B). The dissector is then introduced in the posterior plane at 12 o'clock position, and moved toward the right side to create an adequate posterior separation of the lenticule edge (Figs. 5.6C and D). Once the lenticule edge is separated, the anterior plane is dissected completely till the outer margin of the peripheral ring. The dissection progresses from left to right, and follows "outside-in" movements that reach up to the outer margin of the peripheral ring (Figs. 5.6E and F). This is followed by posterior plane dissection through the pocket created initially in the right side (Fig. 5.6G). It is essential to leave small areas of undissected tissue in the periphery to provide counter-traction during lenticule separation from the overlying cap. These areas should be separated toward the end of dissection. The separated lenticule can be easily extracted with either the forceps, or with the dissector by circumferential motions (Fig. 5.6H).

Jacob et al. have also recommended creating two lamellar channels in opposite directions anterior and posterior to the lenticule in cases with thin lenticules.[9] Anterior lamellar dissection is done first, followed by central posterior lamellar dissection. A thin peripheral rim is left undissected. The lenticule side cut along with the peripheral rim is dissected last in a sequential segmental manner. The lenticule is fixated during the terminal dissection and short circumferential strokes are employed to ensure a smooth and complete dissection of the posterior lamellar cut. The lenticule is then extracted with a microforceps.

Zhao et al. described a "*continuous curvilinear lenticulerrhexis*" technique to directly tear and extract the lenticule from the stromal bed in a continuous circumferential manner without performing lamellar separation.[10] The procedure was observed to be safe and effective in the learning curve; however, it may lead to ripping of the lenticule and retained lenticule fragments, especially in cases with low myopia and resultant thin lenticules. The technique is contraindicated in cases with OBL formation or uneven laser scanning.

Kim et al. described *"Chung's swing technique"*, wherein the posterior lenticule plane is separated first followed by the anterior plane.[11] Once the posterior interface is separated, the anterior interface of the lenticule is identified by lifting and swinging the spatula tip at the left end of the incision and separated into a fan shape. The lenticule is grasped with a McPherson forceps at 12 o'clock, pushed toward the center of the cornea and pulled, in order to remove the lenticule in a clockwise direction. The lenticule is not separated at the 12 o'clock to 3 o'clock and the 8 o'clock to 11 o'clock positions in order to avoid damage by forceps during lenticule extraction. The technique has the advantage of lower operation times; however, an increased incidence of incisional edge tearing may be present.

Hamed et al. described the *"push-up"* and *"push-down"* techniques with a special instrument devised with a Y-shaped tip.[12] In the *"push-up"* technique, the Y-shaped instrument is inserted through the side-cut to push-up the lenticule edge in order to facilitate its visualization. The *"push-down"* technique is useful in cap-lenticular adhesions wherein the Y-shaped instrument is used to engage the lenticule edge and push it down in order to create space for the dissector to enter the anterior plane.

Postoperative Regimen

Postoperatively, topical antibiotics, steroids and lubricating drops are prescribed. We prefer to prescribe topical moxifloxacin (0.5%) three times a day and topical corticosteroids (prednisolone 1%) four times a day, slowly tapered over a period of one month. Topical lubricants are prescribed for 8–12 weeks.

Follow-up examinations are undertaken at 1 day, 1 week, 4 weeks, 3 months, 6 months and 1 year, followed by yearly examinations.

SURGICAL INSTRUMENTS

Various lamellar dissectors and microforceps have been designed to facilitate smooth lenticule dissection and easy extraction (Fig. 5.7).[12-14]

- *SMILE lamellar dissectors*: SMILE lamellar dissectors may be single-ended or double-ended instruments. The single-ended instruments have a thin blunt shaft. The double-ended instruments have an elongated Sinskey-like hook at one end and a thin blunt shaft at the other end (Figs. 5.8A to C). The elongated hook aids in opening the side cut incision. It also facilitates identification of the lenticule edge and the initial delineation of the anterior and posterior lenticule planes. The blunt end may be a thin flat shaft or have an oval spoon-like flattened end, and is used for the

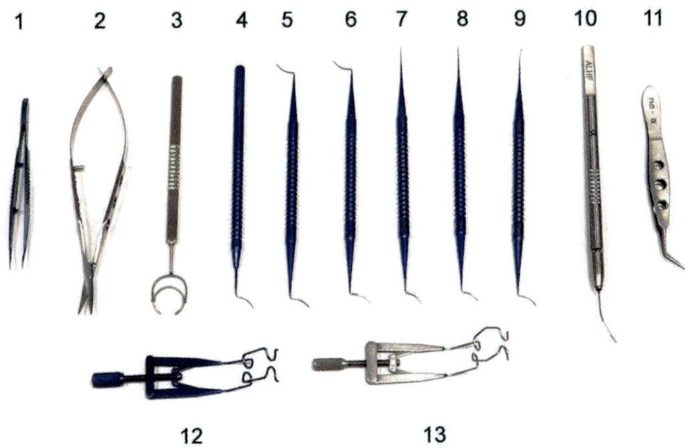

1 Lims forceps
2 Conjunctival scissors
3 Globe fixation ring
4 Lamellar dissector (single-ended)
5,6 Lenticule strippers
7-9 Lamellar dissectors (double-ended)
10 Squeeze-handle microforceps
11 Straight-handle microforceps
12, 13 Self-retaining wire speculum

Fig. 5.7: Surgical instruments used during small incision lenticule extraction (SMILE).

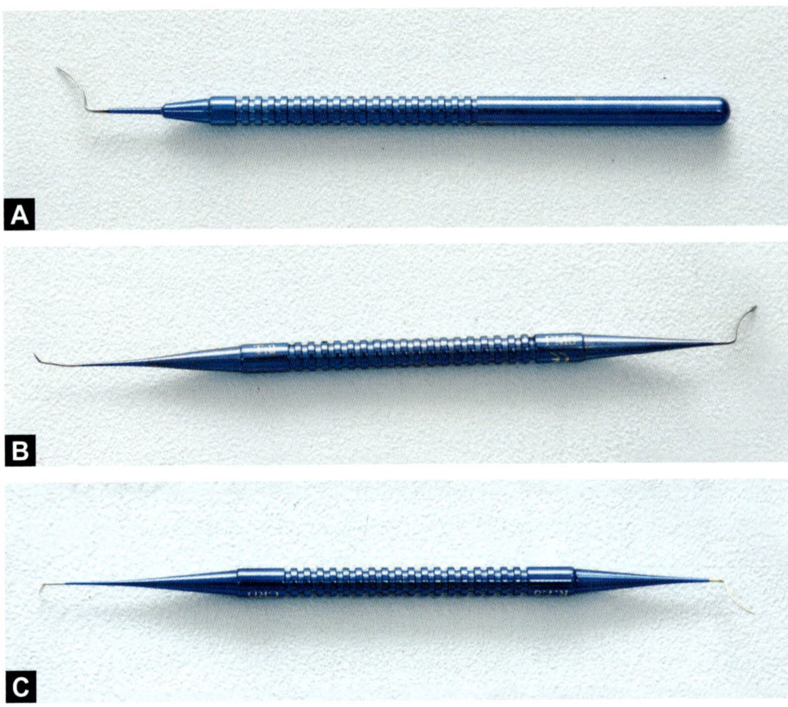

Figs. 5.8A to C: Lamellar dissectors. (A) One-ended lamellar dissector with thin blunt shaft; (B) Lamellar dissector with thin elongated hook at one end and spoon-shaped blunt shaft at the other end; and (C) Lamellar dissector with thin elongated hook at one end and thin blunt shaft at other end.

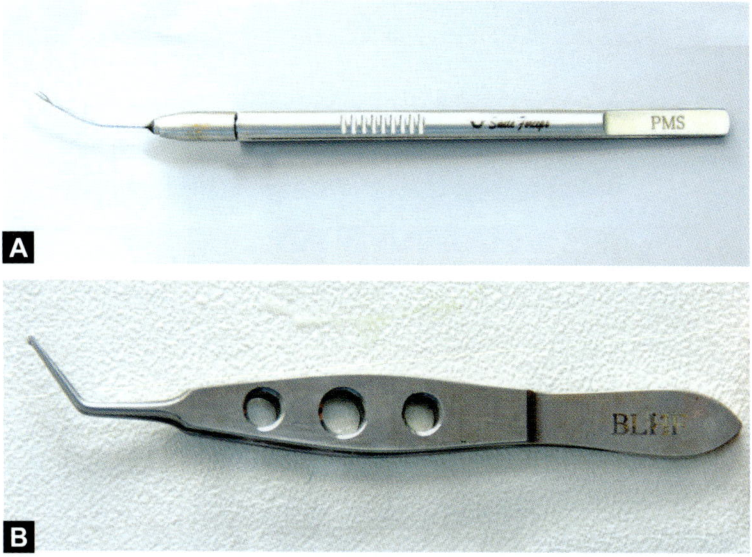

Figs. 5.9A and B: Microforceps for lenticule extraction. (A) 23 gauge squeeze-handled microforceps and (B) Straight handled forceps with blunt texturized tips.

lamellar separation of the lenticule. Its thin shaft reduces risk of incision extension and is angulated to fit the corneal curvature. Examples include Tan Femto Lamellar/SMILE Dissector (ASICO, catalog no. AE-2337), Jod Mehta SMILE/Pocket Dissector (ASICO, catalog no. AE-2403) and SMILE double-ended dissector with spoon tip (Duckworth & Kent Ltd., product no. 6-836).

- *SMILE forceps*: SMILE microforceps are used to extract the lenticule after it has been separated from the stromal bed (Figs. 5.9A and B). The microforceps can either be squeeze-handled or straight-handled. The squeeze-handled microforceps are a modification of retinal membrane peeling forceps used to grasp and extract the lenticule. They have delicate serrated jaws with blunt tip to facilitate easy lenticule removal. Examples include Shah forceps (Segal optics) and Tan EndoGlide forceps (Angio-Tech/Network Medical Products, catalog no. 53-951).

  The second type of forceps includes angled, stainless steel instruments with a flat handle. The tip is thin and may be texturized to allow efficient grasping and extraction of the lenticule while minimizing the risk of incision-extension and tears. Examples include Kelman-McPherson fragment forceps (Geuder) and Stodulka ReLEx SMILE forceps (Rumex International Co., catalog no. 4-2012S).
- *SMILE epithelial/lenticule remover*: It is used to remove the epithelium in cases of accidental epithelial implantation into the SMILE pocket. It has a hook at one end to help the surgeon to extract the edge of lenticule

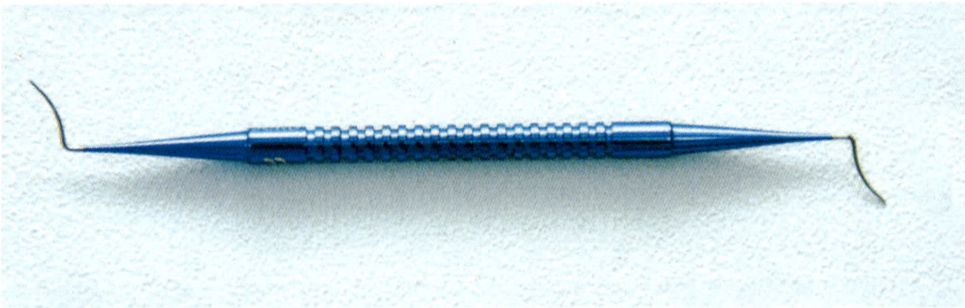

Fig. 5.10: Lenticule stripper.

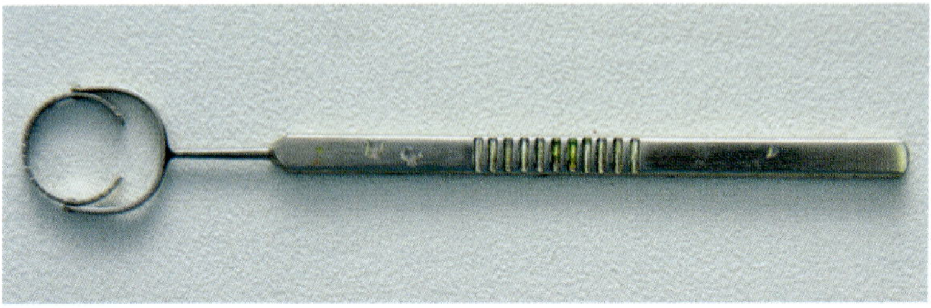

Fig. 5.11: Fixation ring.

with a curved spoon on the other end to allow safe removal of epithelium. It is commercially available as the Jod Mehta SMILE Epithelial/Lenticule Remover (ASICO, catalog no. AE-2404).

- *Y-shaped instrument*: An instrument with a Y-shaped tip (Bechert Nucleus Rotator, product no. E4937, Storz Ophthalmics) may be used to help in the identification of the lenticule edge, as described in the "*push-up*" technique.[12] It may also be used in cases with cap-lenticular adhesions to nudge down the lenticule edge and create a space for the lamellar dissector, as described in the "*push-down*" technique.
- *SMILE lenticule strippers*: Lenticule strippers are useful in cases with cap-lenticular adhesions as a result of inadvertent posterior dissection first (Fig. 5.10).[14] They are inserted into the plane between the posterior surface of the lenticule and underlying stroma, and can be used to hook or pull out the lenticule directly.
- *Fixation ring*: An open fixation ring may be employed to stabilize the globe and prevent inadvertent eye movements during surgery (Fig. 5.11). It is available in various sizes ranging from 13 mm to 16 mm.
- *Lims corneoscleral forceps*: It is a fine toothed forceps used to grasp the conjunctiva and stabilize the globe during lenticule dissection and extraction (Fig. 5.12).
- *Universal wire speculum*: A universal lightweight wire speculum made of stainless steel or titanium is used to separate the eyelids (Fig. 5.13). A self-retaining speculum should be used.

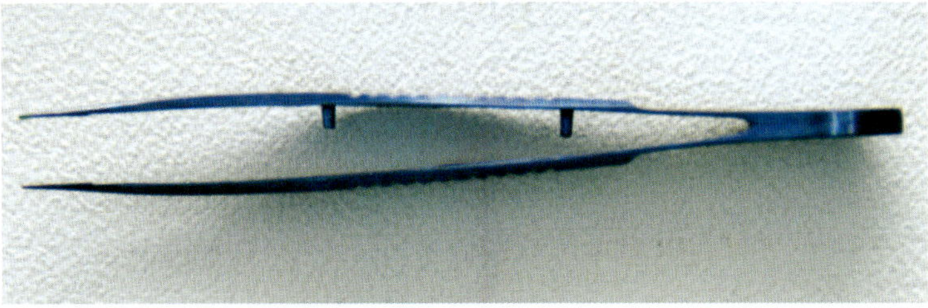

Fig. 5.12: Lims' corneoscleral forceps.

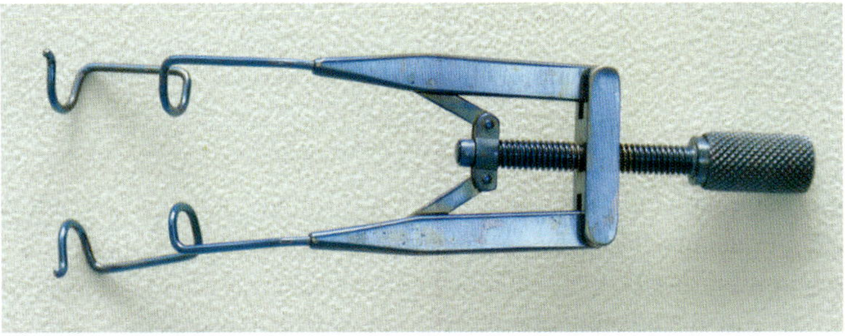

Fig. 5.13: Universal wire speculum.

CONCLUSION

The surgical technique of SMILE is more difficult than conventional flap-based corneal ablative procedures. Preoperative preparation and patient counseling followed by stepwise completion of the procedure can help to ensure a smooth and successful surgery. Modifications of the conventional technique have been developed to facilitate easy lenticule dissection and extraction. Specialized instruments are available for smooth lamellar separation and extraction while minimizing the peripheral tissue damage.

REFERENCES

1. Vetter JM, Faust M, Gericke A, et al. Intraocular pressure measurements during flap preparation using 2 femtosecond lasers and 1 microkeratome in human donor eyes. J Cataract Refract Surg. 2012;38:2011-8.
2. Ang M, Chaurasia SS, Angunawela RI, et al. Femtosecond lenticule extraction (FLEx): clinical results, interface evaluation, and intraocular pressure variation. Invest Ophthalmol Vis Sci. 2012;53:1414-21.
3. Sekundo W, Kunert KS, Blum M. Small incision corneal refractive surgery using the small incision lenticule extraction (SMILE) procedure for the correction of myopia and myopic astigmatism: results of a 6 month prospective study. Br J Ophthalmol. 2011;95:335-9.
4. Shah R, Shah S, Sengupta S. Results of small incision lenticule extraction: All-in-one femtosecond laser refractive surgery. J Cataract Refract Surg. 2011;37:127-37.

5. Shah R, Shah S. Effect of scanning patterns on the results of femtosecond laser lenticule extraction refractive surgery. J Cataract Refract Surg. 2011;37:1636-47.
6. Riau AK, Angunawela RI, Chaurasia SS, et al. Effect of different femtosecond laser-firing patterns on collagen disruption during refractive lenticule extraction. J Cataract Refract Surg. 2012;38:1467-75.
7. Jacob S, Nariani A, Figus M, et al. White ring sign for uneventful lenticule separation in small-incision lenticule extraction. J Cataract Refract Surg. 2016;42:1251-4.
8. Shetty R, Negalur N, Shroff R, et al. Cap lenticular adhesion during small incision lenticular extraction surgery: Causative factors and outcomes. Asia Pac J Ophthalmol (Phila). 2017;6:233-7.
9. Jacob S, Agarwal A, Mazzotta C, et al. Sequential segmental terminal lenticular side-cut dissection for safe and effective small-incision lenticule extraction in thin lenticules. J Cataract Refract Surg. 2017;43:443-8.
10. Zhao Y, Li M, Yao P, et al. Development of the continuous curvilinear lenticulerrhexis technique for small incision lenticule extraction. J Refract Surg. 2015;31:16-21.
11. Kim BK, Mun SJ, Lee DG, et al. Chung's swing technique: A new technique for small-incision lenticule extraction. BMC Ophthalmol. 2016;16:154.
12. Hamed A, Fekry A. Refractive small-incision lenticule extraction: push-up and push-down techniques. J Cataract Refract Surg. 2016;42:1713-5.
13. Liu YC, Mehta JS. Surgical instruments for small incision lenticule extraction (SMILE). Expert Rev Ophthalmol. 2016;11:171-2.
14. Liu YC, Pujara T, Mehta JS. New instruments for lenticule extraction in small incision lenticule extraction (SMILE). PLoS One. 2014;9:e113774.

Chapter

6

Stepwise Approach for Beginners: Navigating the Learning Curve

Anubha Rathi, Manpreet Kaur, Jeewan S Titiyal

INTRODUCTION

In the era of modern refractive surgery, *small incision lenticule extraction (SMILE)* is gaining popularity over corneal ablative procedures for its novelty and favorable outcomes. With spreading awareness and popularity of the procedure, an increasing number of refractive surgeons are transitioning from the conventional flap-based corneal ablative procedures to flap-less refractive lenticule extraction. This leap from flap to cap has not been an easy one, and there is a significant learning curve associated with SMILE.[1] The patient outcome depends on the phase of learning curve of the surgeon.[2] A stepwise approach to this novel surgical procedure will familiarize the surgeon with the unique technical and surgical aspects of the procedure, as well as ensure optimal visual and anatomical outcomes. In this chapter, the various preparative procedures that will help the surgeon to gain familiarity with the procedure are discussed. Video-assisted practical tips are highlighted to facilitate step-by-step lenticule dissection and extraction.

STEPWISE APPROACH DURING THE LEARNING CURVE

The ideal learning curve of any surgical approach is expected to have a smooth rise with easy steps and no sudden leap. However, SMILE has a steep learning curve, even for surgeons experienced in femtosecond laser-assisted in situ keratomileusis (FS-LASIK).[3,4] It is all the more difficult for novice surgeons. In a retrospective study to analyze the learning curve of a novice surgeon, it was observed that an experience of at least 80 eyes is required in order to consistently perform a unilateral SMILE procedure in less than 5 minutes.[1]

A stepwise approach is recommended to ease the tedious learning curve associated with SMILE (Fig. 6.1 and Table 6.1).

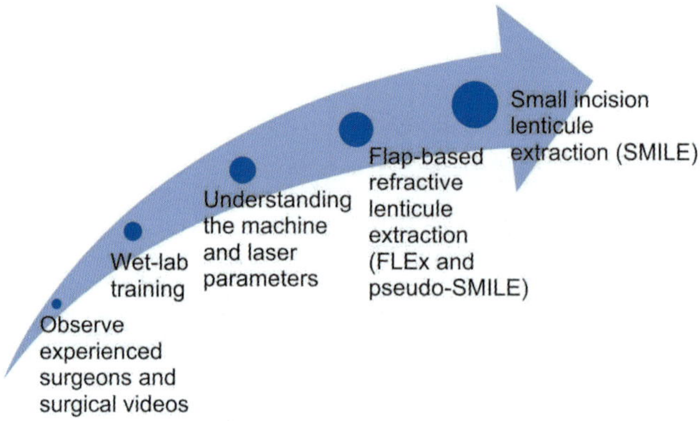

Fig. 6.1: Stepwise learning curve of small incision lenticule extraction.

Table 6.1: Stepwise approach to ease the learning curve of small incision lenticule extraction (SMILE)

Steps	***Procedure***
Observe first	▪ Observe experienced surgeons ▪ Attend live demonstrations ▪ Undertake short-term fellowships
Wet lab training	▪ Tactile feel of the dissection planes and the lenticule ▪ Improved depth perception and identification of dissection planes ▪ Effective handling of the thin refractive lenticule
Flap-based refractive lenticule extraction (21)	FLEx ⟶ pseudo-SMILE ▪ Initial surgical familiarity of the "flap" ▪ Accustoms one to the machine dynamics ▪ Experience in dissecting and extracting the refractive lenticule
Small incision lenticule extraction (1 to 10)	▪ *Understanding the machine and laser parameters* • Check ambient temperature, humidity, and last servicing date • Customize laser and treatment parameters ▪ *Patient selection* • Patient counseling and written informed consent, explain procedure Avoid anxious and hyperactive patients • Anatomical considerations—avoid deep set eyes and narrow palpebral apertures • Magnitude of refractive error—avoid very low refractive errors (thinner lenticule, difficult to identify and remove) ▪ *Surgical technique* • Check instruments, avoid broken/sharp instruments • Identification of lenticule edge • Correct order of lamellar dissection—anterior followed by posterior • Avoid pulling out the lenticule with force, ensure adequate separation before attempting removal • Know when to stop and ask for help!

Observe First

No procedure is learnt in a day. It is important to observe experienced surgeons perform the surgery first. At this stage, attending live demonstrations and undertaking short-term fellowships may be helpful in understanding the numerous surgical steps. The laser parameters, surgical instruments and the technique of lenticule dissection and extraction should be carefully observed to understand the intricacies of the surgical procedure.

Wet-lab Training

For a novice surgeon, a significant number of wet-lab sessions are needed before beginning any refractive surgery. Prior wet-lab training helps to ease the flap-to-cap transition and enables the surgeons to get the tactile feel of the dissection planes and the lenticule. It will help the surgeons to identify the depth of dissection and impart confidence in handling the thin refractive lenticule without damaging the surrounding corneal stroma. SMILE is effectively a closed chamber procedure wherein the entire surgical manipulation is undertaken through a small 2–5 mm incision. This is in stark contrast to FS-LASIK, which entails simply lifting a flap with minimal surgical manipulations thereafter. The quantum leap from LASIK to SMILE requires surgical finesse and experience of lamellar dissection. Wet-lab training goes a long way in helping surgeons to bridge the gap with significant ease (Figs. 6.2A to C).

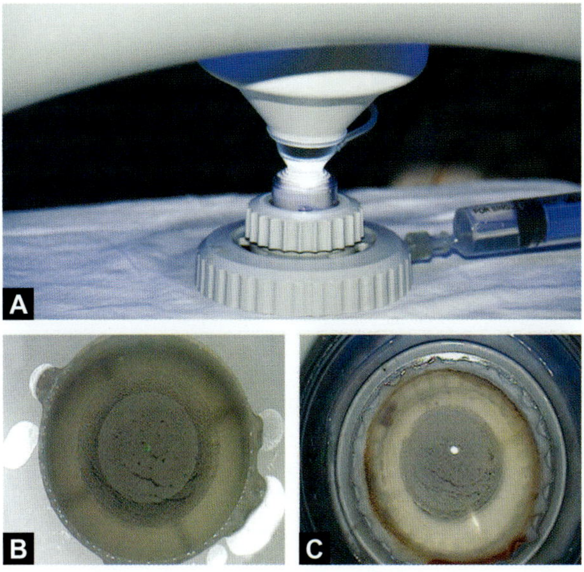

Figs. 6.2A to C: Wet-lab training for refractive lenticule extraction. (A) Experimental grade donor cornea is mounted on an artificial chamber and docked. (B) Femtosecond laser delivery to create intrastromal lenticule. (C) Refractive lenticule can be dissected and extracted from the donor cornea mounted on an artificial chamber.

Orientation with the Machine

Small incision lenticule extraction involves creation of a refractive lenticule using ZEISS VisuMax (Carl Zeiss Meditec, Jena, Germany) femtosecond laser system. Unlike femtosecond LASIK module, there is a single workstation with no excimer laser station. Understanding the machine and its components is of prime importance and has been discussed in Chapter 4 "Understanding the Machine and Laser Settings".

Femtosecond Lenticule Extraction

VisuMax femtosecond laser system was introduced in 2007 mainly for femtosecond lenticule extraction (FLEx).[5] In refractive lenticule extraction (ReLEx) FLEx, femtosecond laser creates an intrastromal corneal lenticule which is removed after creation of a corneal flap (21). It is advisable to begin with FLEx as this gives the surgeons the initial surgical familiarity of the "flap" and also accustoms them to the machine dynamics (Figs. 6.3A to D). Flap-based lenticule extraction simplifies the further surgical manipulations. The surgeon only has to identify the posterior lenticule plane

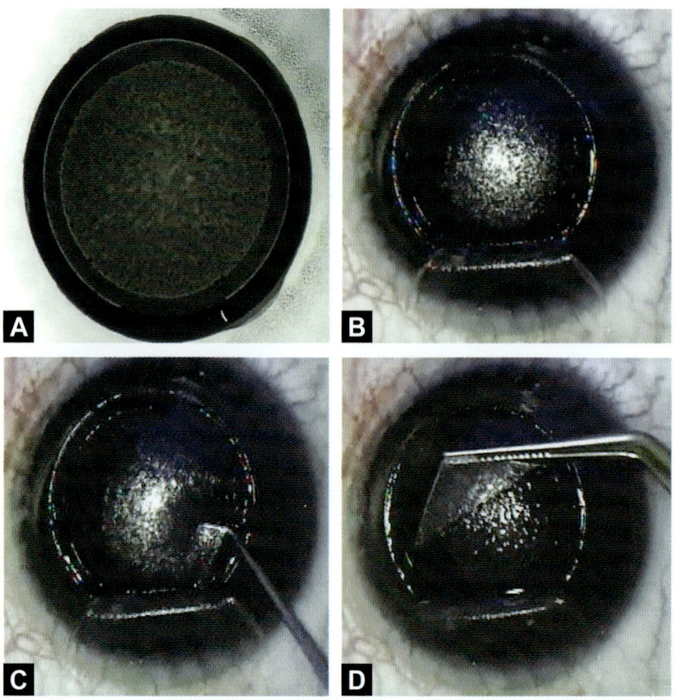

Figs. 6.3A to D: Femtosecond lenticule extraction. (A) Femtosecond laser application to create flap and intrastromal lenticule. (B) Flap is lifted off with Seibel spatula. (C) Lenticule is dissected from stromal bed with elongated hook. (D) Lenticule is grasped with forceps and peeled off from the stromal bed.

after lifting the flap, and also gains experience in dissecting and extracting the refractive lenticule.

Pseudo-Small Incision Lenticule Extraction

A pseudo-SMILE procedure may be performed during the transition phase from FLEx to SMILE (Figs. 6.4A to D). It involves femtosecond laser-assisted creation of an intrastromal lenticule similar to FLEx (📹 21). The laser and treatment parameters are similar to FLEx, with a variation in the hinge position, which is shifted from its initial superior position to the right in order to provide a superior opening for lenticule extraction. The hinge width may be increased to maximum, in order to minimize the circumference of flap-cut.

However, during lenticule dissection and extraction, the flap is not lifted. Instead, a small incision (width 5–6 mm) is opened, and further manipulations including lenticule extraction are undertaken through this incision in a closed chamber manner akin to SMILE.

Pseudo-SMILE serves as an intermediary procedure during the transition from FLEx to SMILE, as it allows the surgeon to practice lenticule extraction

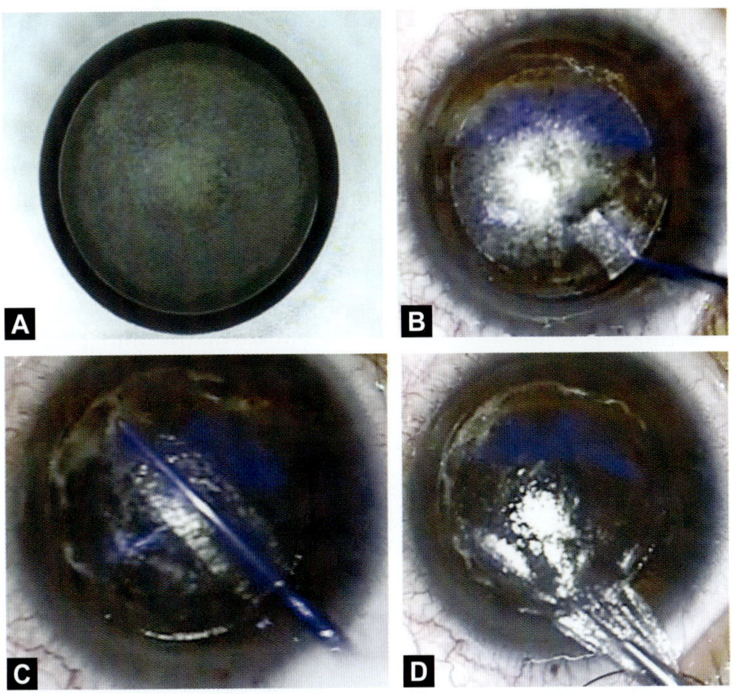

Figs. 6.4A to D: Pseudo-small incision lenticule extraction. (A) Femtosecond laser application to create flap (increased hinge width, position shifted away from superior) and intrastromal lenticule. (B) Small 4–5 mm incision opened superotemporally, without lifting the flap. (C) Anterior and posterior lenticule plane dissected through the small incision. (D) Lenticule grasped with forceps and extracted through the small incision.

through a small incision, with the safety fall-back of an already created flap in case the attempts are not successful.[6]

TAKING THE LEAP: SMALL INCISION LENTICULE EXTRACTION

Small incision lenticule extraction involves creation of an intrastromal lenticule and its extraction from a small side incision (1 to 10). It is more challenging than flap-based corneal ablative procedures. After a reasonable number of observations, wet-lab sessions and FLEx, a surgeon may confidently move to actually cracking the SMILE!

Handling the Machine, Treatment and Laser Parameters

- *Get oriented with the machine, check ambient temperature, humidity and last date of servicing*
  A surgeon already familiar with the machine finds it easier to perform the surgery. Wet-lab training and experience of FLEx helps in this regard. Most importantly, the machine must be in good working condition, adequately serviced and functioning at a room temperature of around 18–25°C and ambient humidity of 30–70%.[7] Understanding the bed control, joystick movement, suction button as well as the laser footswitch is important and is usually dealt with during the wet-lab training.
- *Laser parameters: Before hitting the laser button!*
  It is advisable to recheck all the treatment parameters before starting the surgery.

  Laser settings depend on the mode selected. The "*standard mode*" incorporates the set manufacturer recommended settings. For beginners, the authors advise performing the surgery under *expert mode* wherein the settings may be modified as per ease. For the initial cases, it is advisable to keep the energy levels in the range of 30–34 nJ to ensure complete cuts with no adhesions. These levels should be brought down to 28–30 nJ later as the surgeon gains more competence, as it has been seen that higher energy levels may lead to suboptimal visual recovery and may lengthen the recovery time of patients undergoing SMILE.[8]

  The usual settings preferred by the authors are summarized in Table 6.2.
  - *Spot distance (1 step = 0.10 μm)*: Recommended 4.5 μm for lenticule and cap, 2.0 μm for lenticule and cap side-cut.
  - *Track distance (1 step = 0.10 μm)*: Recommended 4.5 μm for lenticule and cap, 2.0 μm for lenticule and cap side-cut.
  - *Energy (1 step = 5 nJ)*: Around 30–34 for beginners (total energy 150–170 nJ).
  - *Scan direction (spiral in; spiral out)*: Spiral in for posterior plane, spiral out for anterior plane (fixed).

Table 6.2: Customized laser and treatment parameters for beginners in small incision lenticule extraction

Laser parameters		***Treatment parameters***	
Spot distance	▪ 4.5 µm for lenticule and cap ▪ 2.0 µm for lenticule and cap side cut	*Cap cut*	▪ Thickness 120 µm ▪ Diameter 1 mm more than lenticule diameter
Track distance	▪ 4.5 µm for lenticule and cap ▪ 2.0 µm for lenticule and cap side cut	*Cap side-cut*	▪ Width 4–5 mm ▪ Number of incisions one or two ▪ Incision position 110°
Energy offset	▪ 30–34 (total energy 150–170 nJ) ▪ Titrate energy to achieve uniform bubble layer with minimal opaque bubble layer and adhesions	*Lenticule cut*	▪ Diameter 6–7 mm ▪ Transition zone 0.10 for CYL, 0 for SPH ▪ Minimum lenticule thickness 15–30 µm
Scan direction	▪ Spiral in for posterior plane ▪ Spiral out for anterior plane	*Lenticule side cut*	▪ Lenticule side cut angle 90–135°
Preferred mode	▪ Expert (modifiable parameters)		

- *Mode*: The expert mode should be selected as the parameters are modifiable in this mode as per surgeon expertise and stage of learning.

▪ *Treatment parameters for beginners*

A beginner may find the lamellar nature of SMILE surgery difficult to perform in the initial phase. The treatment parameters may be modified to ease the subsequent surgical steps. The lenticule-cap disparity should be set at the maximum limit of 1 mm, as it helps in the easy identification of the lenticule edge and subsequent dissection. A wider cap side-cut incision of 4-5 mm allows enough room for movement of instruments while dissecting the planes and extracting the lenticule. The minimum thickness of the lenticule is usually kept as 15 µm. This is the peripheral thickness of the lenticule and may be increased to 25-30 µm for initial cases to ease the lenticule edge identification. The central thickness of the refractive lenticule is based on the refractive error of the eye and is calculated as per standard nomogram by the machine. On an average, for every diopter of refractive error to be corrected, around 13 µm of tissue is removed.

- *Cap thickness*: 120 µm
- *Cap diameter:* 7-8 mm (1 mm over lenticule diameter)

- *Lenticule diameter:* 6–7 mm (based on the mesopic pupil size)
- *Cap side-cut*: 4–5 mm, may use two side cuts instead of one
- *Minimum thickness of lenticule*: 15 µm for higher refractive errors, 25–30 µm for lower refractive errors.

Patient Selection

For any surgeon beginning with a new surgical approach, more than anything else a "patient" patient is required. The counseling at this stage is of paramount importance.

- *Patient counseling*

  A written informed consent must be taken. The patient should be explained the steps of the procedure in brief, as well as what is expected from the patient during the surgery. Hyperactive and over anxious patients should ideally be avoided in the initial phase of learning curve.
- *Anatomical considerations*

  Avoid very deep set eyes and those with narrow palpebral apertures as they may be associated with intraoperative suction loss, decentration and difficult docking. Such complications may be difficult to handle in the hands of a beginner.
- *Magnitude of refractive error*

  The dimensions and thickness of the refractive lenticule depend on the amount of refractive error to be treated. On an average, for every diopter of refractive error to be corrected, around 13 µm of tissue is removed.[9] For initial cases, it is advisable for surgeon to begin with higher refractive errors wherein a thicker lenticule is expected. Such a lenticule can be easily delineated at the time of dissection and held with forceps at the time of removal, with lesser chance of tearing. Also, patients with higher refractive errors have been seen to be more adjusting with slower visual recovery which may be associated with the learning curve of a SMILE surgeon.

Surgical Technique

The surgical technique for SMILE has been described in detail in Chapter 5 "Surgical Technique of Small Incision Lenticule Extraction". We have highlighted the salient points that the beginner must keep in mind to ensure a smooth surgery (1 to 10).

- *Patient position and preparation*

  Before starting the surgery, the patient should be made comfortable and counseled for the procedure. The bed is moved to the patient shifting position. The patient is made to lie down supine with the head placed in the head ring to avoid inadvertent head movement during docking which could lead to untimely suction loss. The bed is then moved in the observation position beneath the surgical microscope. Self-retaining light-weight speculum should be used to ensure adequate exposure.

- *Docking and centration*

  The size of the treatment pack varies with the white-to-white (WTW) measurement of the patient's eye. In standard cases with WTW around 10–12 mm, the size is usually small (S). Choosing the right treatment pack size is important to ensure a good suction. A larger pack size may lead to inadvertent suction loss during the procedure and lead to suboptimal outcome and may impede the surgery.

  The patient should be asked to fixate on the green light while docking. The surgeon should ensure a clean contact glass, as interface debris may lead to the formation of black spots and opaque bubble layer which will make the subsequent dissection more difficult.

  The corneal surface should be adequately moist, with no pooling of fluid or dry spots.

  It is important to note that the bed should be moved up slowly during centration till the contact glass interface touches the cornea. Adequate centration should be ensured while docking. The treatment is centered on the coaxially sighted corneal light reflex which is the reflection of the blinking green light on the cornea, and is aligned with the visual axis of the patient. The visual axis of the patient is centered to the vertex of the contact glass, which is in turn centered on the laser system and decides the center of the lenticule to be created. In patients with small to moderate angle kappa, this may be a better tool for centration as compared to the eye tracker in FS-LASIK, which depends on the effective pupil center.[10]

  Once the docking is complete, the top button on the joystick is pressed to create suction. Conjunctiva should not be entrapped between the contact lens and ocular surface as it may lead to untimely suction loss.

  After suction is created, the infrared centration check should be done which highlights the pupil. In case of any doubt, repeat docking may be done. Even in the early phase of the learning curve, SMILE has been observed to achieve accurate centration and good postoperative visual outcomes.[11,12]

- *Laser cuts*

  Once centration is ensured, the surgeon hits the laser pedal, which has to be pressed continuously till the treatment is completed. The progress of treatment can be visualized on the screen output at all times.

- *Dissection of the cleavage planes*

  The patient is shifted to the observation end of the machine for lenticule dissection and extraction.

  Lenticule edge identification is the initial and most important step. At the beginning of surgical dissection, margin of the lenticule is well demarcated and can be easily made out but may get camouflaged later due to multiple attempts of dissection. Hence, it is important to hit the right plane at this stage itself! The hooked end of the dissection spatula is used to open the incision. It is advisable not to open the complete incision in one go. The left half of the incision may be opened with the hooked instrument dissecting the anterior cleavage plane and the right half of the incision may be initially opened with the hooked instrument in the posterior dissection plane (Figs. 6.5A to C). This delineates the planes well before attempting further dissection.

The anterior interface is dissected first with a dissector that is introduced into the plane through the left end of the side incision. Complete dissection must be done ensuring no residual adhesion to reduce the possibility of a retained lenticule later. Then the posterior interface is dissected with the dissector.

The posterior plane must never be dissected out first as it is very difficult to separate the anterior plane after posterior plane dissection due to lack of a posterior support. During dissection of posterior plane,

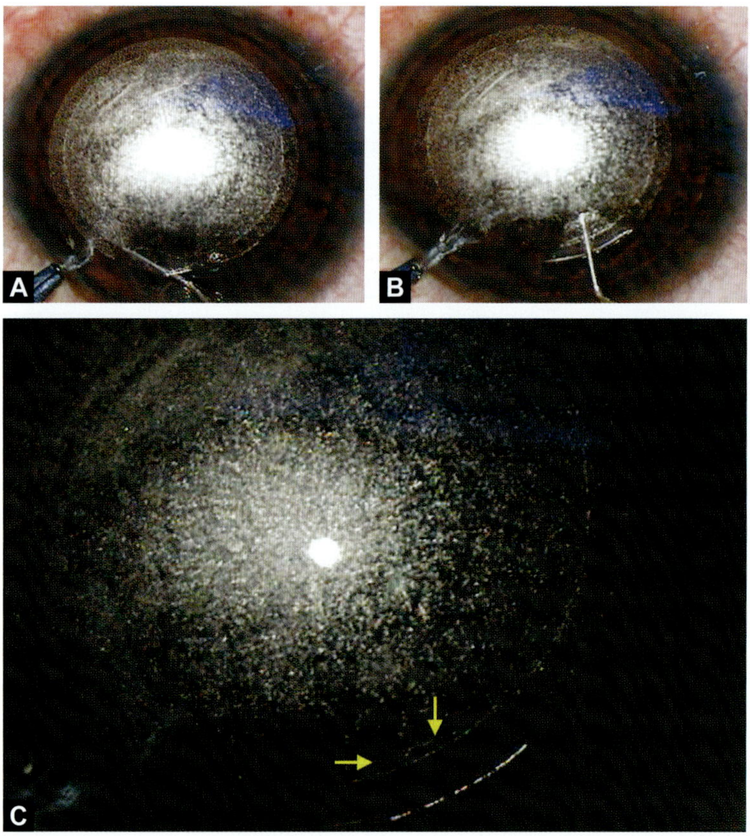

Figs. 6.5A to C: Lenticule edge identification. (A) Left half of the incision opened with the hooked instrument dissecting the anterior cleavage plane. (B) Right half of the incision opened with the hooked instrument dissecting the posterior cleavage plane. (C) Lenticule edge identified (arrows: Lenticule edge).

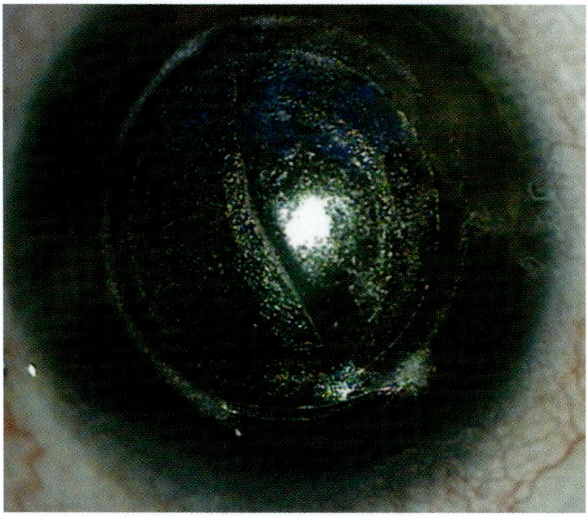

Fig. 6.6: Lenticule folded in half to facilitate easy extraction by a microforceps.

few peripheral areas must be allowed to remain undissected till the end to provide counter-traction for completing dissection.

The lenticule may be folded on one side to ensure visibility and give a firm hold at the time of removal (Fig. 6.6). The refractive lenticule is removed using a nontoothed forceps. Even at this stage, smooth circumferential removal should be done similar to performing a capsulorrhexis. No forceful pulling should be attempted to prevent tearing of lenticule or damage to the posterior cornea.

The lenticule must be examined for completeness after extraction, to rule out any retained fragments. Various complications may occur during the initial phase, which may be effectively managed as detailed in Chapter 8 "Intraoperative Complications in Small Incision Lenticule Extraction".

Knowing When to Stop!!!

It is important to know what to do but more important to know what ***NOT*** to do and where to stop! In this respect, a surgeon beginning with SMILE must remember that the patient should never suffer because of the learning curve of the surgery as such. Over enthusiastic dissection should be avoided to prevent any permanent damage to the cornea. Ask for timely help whenever there is a need. Initial cases must be done under expert guidance. Almost all possible complications that may occur during the learning phase can be managed effectively if a surgeon abandons the procedure well in time whenever things go out of hand. Every doctor is taught in the infancy of their medical training to cause *NO HARM* and make the treatment a part of the cure, *NOT* the problem. We must all abide by this golden rule at all times!

CONCLUSION

The learning curve of SMILE is tedious but manageable. Making the flap-to-cap transition is a surgical challenge even for FS-LASIK experienced surgeons. The visual and anatomical outcomes vary with the stage of the learning curve of the surgeon. Hence, a stepwise approach is recommended for easing the transition from flap to cap. This includes observation, wet-lab training, beginning with FLEx and pseudo-SMILE, customizing treatment parameters and laser settings along with proper case selection. All these together aid the surgeon in effectively cracking the SMILE!!

REFERENCES

1. Pradhan K, Reinstein D, Carp G, et al. (2013). Learning curve for small incision lenticule extraction (SMILE) of a novice corneal laser refractive surgeon evaluated by procedure time for consecutive cases. European Society of Cataract & Refractive Surgeons. [online] ESCRS website. Available from http://escrs.org/amsterdam2013/programme/free-papers-details.asp?id=15825&day=0 [Accessed October 2013].
2. Taneri S, Kießler S, Rost A, et al. [Experience with Introduction of SMILE: Learning Phase of our First 200 Treatments]. Klin Monbl Augenheilkd. 2017;234:70-76.
3. Ramirez-Miranda A, Ramirez-Luquin T, Navas A, et al. Refractive lenticule extraction complications. Cornea. 2015;34(Suppl 10):S65-7.
4. Titiyal JS, Kaur M, Rathi A, et al. Learning curve of small incision lenticule extraction: challenges & complications. Cornea. 2017 Aug 9. [Epub ahead of print]
5. Sekundo W, Kunert K, Russmann C, et al. First efficacy and safety study of femtosecond lenticule extraction for the correction of myopia. J Cataract Refract Surg. 2008;34:1513-20.
6. Ang M, Mehta JS, Chan C, et al. Refractive lenticule extraction: transition and comparison of 3 surgical techniques. J Cataract Refract Surg. 2014;40(9):1415-24.
7. VisuMax. VisuMax Femtosecond System. [online] ZEISS website. Available from: https://www.zeiss.com/meditec/int/products/ophthalmology-optometry/cornea-refractive/laser-treatment/femtosecond-laser-solutions/visumax.html#technical-data [Accessed March 2017].
8. Ji YW, Kim M, Kang DSY, et al. Lower laser energy levels lead to better visual recovery after small-incision lenticule extraction: prospective randomized clinical trial. Am J Ophthalmol. 2017;179:159-70.
9. Ganesh S, Brar S. Clinical outcomes of small incision lenticule extraction with accelerated cross-linking (ReLEx SMILE Xtra) in patients with thin corneas and borderline topography. J Ophthalmol. 2015;2015:263412.
10. Li M, Zhao J, Miao H, et al. Mild decentration measured by a Scheimpflug camera and its impact on visual quality following SMILE in the early learning curve. Invest Ophthalmol Vis Sci. 2014;55:3886-92.
11. Reinstein DJ, Gobbe M, Gobbe L, et al. Optical zone centration accuracy using corneal fixation-based SMILE compared to eye tracker-based femtosecond laser-assisted lasik for myopia. J Refract Surg. 2015;31(9):586-92.
12. Vestergaard A, Ivarsen AR, Asp S, et al. Small-incision lenticule extraction for moderate to high myopia: predictability, safety, and patient satisfaction. J Cataract Refract Surg. 2012;38(11):2003-10.

Chapter 7

Refractive and Physiological Outcomes of Small Incision Lenticule Extraction

Pranita Sahay, Manpreet Kaur, Jeewan S Titiyal

INTRODUCTION

Refractive lenticule extraction (ReLEx) is a safe and effective refractive procedure for the correction of myopia and myopic astigmatism.[1] Since its introduction in 2006, it has evolved from a flap-based femtosecond lenticule extraction (FLEx) to the present day small incision lenticule extraction (SMILE). The visual and physiological outcomes have improved with evolving technology, and are comparable to femtosecond-laser-assisted in situ keratomileusis (FS-LASIK). Moreover, SMILE has been observed to have superior refractive stability with fewer incidences of postoperative regression, better ocular surface stability as well as biomechanical strength. The expanding refractive applications of SMILE have produced optimal results even in higher degrees of myopia, astigmatism, and hyperopia. In this chapter, the visual outcomes are discussed in detail, in terms of visual acuity as well as the quality of vision and higher-order aberrations (HOAs). The physiological outcomes will be elaborated, with emphasis on tear film stability and biomechanical strength.

REFRACTIVE OUTCOMES

The refractive success of a procedure is measured in terms of both visual acuity as well as quality of vision (Table 7.1).

Visual Acuity

Visual acuity is one of the most important refractive outcomes concerned with patient satisfaction. Safety, efficacy, predictability, and long-term stability of the procedure are assessed in addition to measuring the uncorrected visual acuity.[2-13]

- *Efficacy*: The efficacy of any refractive surgery is defined as the proportion of eyes that achieve an uncorrected distance visual acuity (UDVA) of 20/20 or better. The efficacy of SMILE for achieving UDVA more than 20/20 at 6 months ranges from 62% to 90%, and UDVA more than 20/40 at 6 months varies from 95% to 100% (Table 7.2).

Table 7.1: Refractive and physiological outcomes of small incision lenticule extraction (SMILE)

Visual outcomes	*Results*
Visual acuity	
▪ Efficacy	UDVA > 20/20 ▪ 62–90% at 6 months ▪ High myopia: 85% at 2 years ▪ Low myopia: 96% at 1 year ▪ Low astigmatism: 58% cases ▪ High astigmatism: 38% cases Hyperopia: UDVA > 20/40 is achieved in 87% cases at 3 months
▪ Safety	▪ 0.50% lost more than 2 lines ▪ 0.50% lost 2 lines ▪ 8% lost 1 line ▪ 60% were unchanged ▪ 27% gained 1 line ▪ 4% gained 2 lines
▪ Predictability	Predictability of SMILE for ±0.5 D of residual refractive error ▪ 77–100% in myopes ▪ High myopia: 78–92% ▪ Low myopia: 84–97% ▪ Hyperopia: only 65% cases
▪ Stability	The change in MRSE varies from 0.01 D to 0.1 D In high myopes the myopic regression has been noted to be comparatively high (−0.2 D to −0.36 D)
▪ Visual recovery time	Delayed visual recovery due to the interface haze may be present
Visual quality	
▪ Optical aberrations	Increase in total higher-order aberrations, coma, and spherical aberrations
▪ Contrast sensitivity	Variable results of contrast sensitivity in different studies (increase or decrease or stable)
▪ Corneal clarity	Interface haze observed in the early postoperative period becomes insignificant after 1 year of surgery
Physiological outcomes	
▪ Corneal sensations	Decreases after surgery but recover to its preoperative value by 3–6 months
▪ Tear film changes	Decrease in the OSDI score, TBUT, and tear osmolarity after surgery Gradually recovers, with 80% cases being free of lubricant use at 6 months after surgery
▪ Corneal biomechanical strength	Decrease in corneal biomechanical strength. Decrease in CH and CRF on ORA

(UDVA: Uncorrected distance visual acuity; MRSE: Manifest refraction spherical equivalent; OSDI: Ocular surface disease index; TBUT: Tear film breakup time; CH: Corneal hysteresis; CRF: Corneal resistance factor; ORA: Ocular response analyzer).

Table 7.2: Efficacy of small incision lenticule extraction (SMILE) in myopia and myopic astigmatism

Study	Number of eyes	Follow-up	UDVA > 20/20	UDVA > 20/40
Sekundo et al.[2]	91	6 months	83.5%	97.6%
Kamiya et al.[3]	52	1 year	94%	100%
Shah et al.[4]	51	6 months	62%	95%
Zhao et al.[5]	50	6 months	90%	100%
Vestergaard et al.[6]	246	3 months	–	100%
Lin et al.[7]	61	3 months	58.3%	–
Hjortdal et al.[8]	670	3 months	80.1%	94.2%
Low myopia				
Ganesh et al.[9]	60	3 months	97%	100%
Reinstein et al.[10]	120	1 year	96%	100%
High myopia				
Yıldırım et al.[11]	45	2 years	85%	–
Myopia with astigmatism				
Ivarsen et al.[12]				
Low astigmatism (0.75–2.5 D)	669	3 months	58%	94%
High astigmatism (>2.5 D)	106	3 months	38%	84%

(UDVA: Uncorrected distance visual acuity).

The efficacy of SMILE is less in higher magnitude of refractive errors as well as coexistent astigmatism. In high myopes, a UDVA of 20/20 or better is attained in only 85% cases, while in low myopes, 96% of cases achieve UDVA of 20/20 or better.

The presence of astigmatism adversely affects the visual outcomes, with only 58% cases of myopia and low astigmatism (<2.5 DC) attaining UDVA of 20/20 or better at 3 months. In cases with high astigmatism of more than 2.5 D in magnitude, the visual acuity is further compromised with only 38% cases achieving UDVA of 20/20 or better at 3 months (*see* Table 7.1).

- *Safety*: "Safety" of a procedure is defined as the number of eyes with an unchanged corrected distance visual acuity (CDVA) after the refractive surgery. The safety of SMILE has been proven in various studies, and the results are comparable in different magnitudes of refractive error (Table 7.3). Six months after SMILE, 0.50% cases lost more than two lines of Snellen's visual acuity, 0.50% lost two lines, 8% lost one line, 60% were unchanged, 27% gained one line, and 4% gained two lines.
- *Predictability*: "Predictability" is a measure of the accuracy of the refractive procedure, and is defined as the number of eyes with postoperative

Table 7.3: Safety of small incision lenticule extraction in myopia and myopic astigmatism

Study	*Number of eyes*	*Follow-up*	*Loss of > 2 lines (%)*	*Loss of 2 lines (%)*	*Loss of 1 line (%)*	*No gain or loss (%)*	*Gain of 1 line (%)*	*Gain of ≥ 2 lines (%)*
Sekundo et al.[2]	91	6 months	1	1	9	53	32	3
Kamiya et al.[3]	52	1 year	0	4	17	63	15	0
Shah et al.[4]	39	6 months	0	0	4	70	21	4
Lin et al.[7]	61	3 months	0	3.3	3.3	93.3	0	0
Hjortdal et al.[8]	670	3 months	0	2.3	15	49	30	3.7
Vestergaard et al.[6]	246	3 months	0	0	6	96	24	1
Low myopia								
Ganesh et al.[9]	60	3 months	0	0	0	60	32	8
Reinstein et al.[10]	120	1 year	0	0	9	66	23	2
High myopia								
Yıldırım et al.[11]	45	2 years	0	0	2	60	38	0
Myopia with astigmatism								
Ivarsen et al.[12] ▪ Low astigmatism (0.75–2.5 D) ▪ High astigmatism (>2.5 D)	 669 106	 3 months 3 months	 2.8% 0.9%					

Table 7.4: Predictability of small incision lenticule extraction (SMILE) in myopia and myopic astigmatism

Study	Number of eyes	Follow-up	±0.5 D of emmetropia	±1 D of emmetropia
Sekundo et al.[2]	91	6 months	80.2%	95.6%
Kamiya et al.[3]	52	1 year	100%	100%
Shah et al.[4]	39	6 months	91%	100%
Lin et al.[7]	60	3 months	98.33%	100%
Zhao et al.[5]	50	6 months	92%	98%
Hjortdal et al.[8]	670	3 months	80%	94%
Vestergaard et al.[6]	246	3 months	77%	95%
Low myopia				
Ganesh et al.[9]	60	3 months	97%	–
Reinstein et al.[10]	120	1 year	84%	–
High myopia				
Yıldırım et al.[11]	45	2 years	92%	100%
Pedersen et al.[13]	87	3 years	78%	90%
Myopia with astigmatism				
Ivarsen et al.[12]				
▪ Low astigmatism (0.75–2.5 D)	669	3 months	77%	95%
▪ High astigmatism (>2.5 D)	106	3 months	77%	97%

refraction within ±1.00 D and ±0.5 D of the target. SMILE has been observed to have good predictability, with 77–100% eyes achieving refractive correction within ±0.5 D of the intended target. The predictability varies from 78% to 92% in high myopia and from 84% to 97% in low myopia. Relatively low predictability is observed in astigmatism, with only 77% cases within ±0.5 D of the intended target at 3 months (Table 7.4).

- *Stability*: "Stability" is depicted by the change in the manifest refraction spherical equivalent (MRSE) in the postoperative period. Kamiya et al. observed a change in MRSE by 0.05 ± 0.16 D at the end of 1 year.[3] Pederson et al. observed higher magnitude of myopic regression (–0.36 ± 0.6 D) with increasing magnitude of refractive error (Table 7.5).[13]

The refractive regression after myopia is a result of the wound-healing response after refractive surgery, and is exaggerated in higher magnitude of refractive errors.[14] The wound-healing phase involves keratocyte activation, followed by transformation into myofibroblast cells that contract and contribute to the corneal steepening.[15] Epithelial

Table 7.5: Stability of small incision lenticule extraction in myopia and myopic astigmatism

Study	Number of eyes	Follow-up	MRSE
Kamiya et al.[3]	52	1 year	Δ 0.05 ± 0.16 D
Shah et al.[4]	39	6 months	Δ −0.06 ± 0.27 D
Sekundo et al.[2]	91	6 months	Δ +0.01 D
Low myopia			
Ganesh et al.[9]	60	3 months	−0.15 ± 0.19 D
Reinstein et al.[10]	120	1 year	−0.05 ± 0.36 D
High myopia			
Yıldırım et al.[11]	45	2 years	−0.2 ± 0.56 D
Pedersen et al.[13]	87	3 years	Δ −0.36 ± 0.6 D

(MRSE: Manifest refraction spherical equivalent; Δ: Change in MRSE).

hyperplasia also occurs during the wound-healing phase and leads to an increase in the epithelial thickness in the central and superior part of the cornea. These changes result in corneal steepening and refractive regression post SMILE.[16]

Smaller size of the optical zone, weak corneal biomechanics, low preoperative pachymetry, and low residual stromal bed are the other risk factors that contribute to the postoperative refractive regression.

Visual Recovery Time

A delayed visual recovery has been observed after SMILE, more so in the initial learning curve. Interface haze may develop after SMILE due to surgical manipulations, and has been postulated to contribute to the delayed visual recovery.[17] Higher-frequency femtosecond laser with low-energy settings reduces the irregularity of the interface surface and helps in minimizing the interface haze.[18] The pattern of laser trajectory also affects the visual recovery. Faster recovery is observed when the back of the lenticule is scanned from the periphery to the center and front of the lenticule from center to periphery.[19]

Visual Quality

Quality of vision impacts the patient satisfaction after surgery, and depends upon the HOAs, contrast sensitivity, and corneal clarity. Difficult lenticule dissection during the initial learning curve results in bowman membrane microdistortions, and has been observed to negatively impact the quality of vision.[20] This is a result of the excessive light scattering by an irregular interface.

- *Optical aberrations*: The quality of vision is significantly affected by ocular aberrations.[7] SMILE results in a significant increase in the total HOAs, coma as well as spherical aberrations. A positive correlation has been observed between the amount of refractive error and the induced HOA, with higher refractive error correction inducing more HOAs.[21] This can be explained by the exaggerated wound-healing response that occurs in cases with high refractive error. Also, change in the corneal asphericity from prolate to oblate leads to an increase in the amount of induced spherical aberrations. Sekundo et al. reported an increase in HOA from 0.17 μm to 0.27 μm (Malacara notation) at 1-year follow-up.[22]
- *Contrast sensitivity*: Contrast sensitivity is an important aspect of visual function. Majority of studies have not observed any significant difference after surgery, with similar mesopic and photopic contrast sensitivities.[6,22] An increase in the contrast sensitivity 1 year after SMILE has also been observed for the spatial frequencies of 3, 6, 12, and 18 cycles per degree.[10]

  In contrast, Ganesh et al. reported a decrease in the contrast sensitivity which recovers by the third postoperative month.[23]
- *Corneal clarity*: A transient corneal haze is often observed during the slit lamp examination in the early postoperative period. Corneal haze usually decreases with time and becomes clinically insignificant by the end of 1 year. This is the cause for delayed visual recovery post SMILE. It has been speculated that the corneal haze occurs as a result of deposition of debris in the interface, which subsequently induces an inflammatory response. This correlates with the extent of mechanical manipulation and laser-related collateral tissue damage.

  The back-scattered light intensity from the anterior stroma is increased after SMILE as observed during in-vivo confocal microscopy (IVCM).[24] Scheimpflug corneal densitometry and optical coherence tomography have also been used to quantify corneal opacification by detecting the corneal backscatter.[25,26]

SMALL INCISION LENTICULE EXTRACTION IN HYPEROPIA

Hyperopic correction with SMILE is still in its nascent phase and there is paucity of literature regarding the same. Though hyperopic correction with SMILE is not US-FDA approved, there are few studies that have reported their initial experience with the same.[27,28]

The initial reports have established the safety and efficacy of the procedure, with only 2.1% of eyes losing two lines or more of Snellen's visual acuity at 9 months in a study of 47 hyperopic eyes. A total of 97% cases achieved uncorrected visual acuity of 0.5 or better.[28]

At present, the procedure has low predictability for hyperopia, with only 22% of eyes within 0.50 D of intended correction, and 78% of eyes within 1.00 D of target refraction after 9 months as observed by Sekundo et al.[27] Significant regression is observed in the postoperative period, and a nomogram optimization that aims for initial overcorrection may help to counteract the regression associated with epithelial remodeling.

PHYSIOLOGICAL OUTCOMES

Though refractive outcomes are of paramount importance, physiological outcomes like change in corneal sensations and tear film stability have a great impact on the patient's quality of vision and post-surgical dependence on topical lubricants. SMILE has been observed to have superior biomechanical strength and ocular surface stability as compared to flap-based corneal ablative procedures (Table 7.1).

Corneal Sensations

The presence of intact corneal innervation and sensations is essential to maintain a stable ocular surface with a healthy tear film. Corneal hypoesthesia is observed after all refractive surgeries, but the changes are less prominent after SMILE in view of better preservation of the sub-basal nerve plexus.[29] Denoyer et al. assessed the IVCM changes in corneal nerves post SMILE and observed a decrease in the sub-basal corneal nerve length and density. Fast regeneration of transected corneal nerves is observed, with a return to the preoperative levels by 6 months. Liu et al. measured the sub-basal nerve density on IVCM and observed a decrease from 22.37 ± 2.27 mm/mm^2 preoperatively to 17.40 ± 2.14 mm/mm^2 at 1 week, followed by a gradual recovery to the preoperative levels of 22.93 ± 2.53 mm/mm^2 after 3 months.[30]

As there is less severe nerve denervation, wound repair and nerve regeneration occur more rapidly, leading to early recovery of corneal sensations.[31]

Tear Film Stability

Dry eye is the most common postoperative complication after corneal refractive surgery.[32] It not only causes damage to the ocular surface but also causes symptoms of ocular discomfort associated with visual disturbance. There is a degradation of both the visual outcomes as well as the quality of daily life. Most cases experience mild-to-moderate symptoms of dry eye for the first few months after surgery. Chronic dry eye is observed in 20–40% cases after LASIK which persists even after 6 months.[33]

The pathogenesis of post-refractive surgery dry eye is explained by the transection of sub-basal nerve fibers resulting in corneal hypoesthesia. This decreases the tear film quality by decreasing the tear secretion, blink rate, and epithelial wound healing, resulting in symptoms of dry eye.

The ocular surface disease index (OSDI) score, tear film stability (tear breakup time), and tear osmolarity are impaired after SMILE. However, improvement is noted with time, and 80% of patients undergoing SMILE are free from lubricants after 6 months of surgery.[34]

Corneal Biomechanical Strength

Post-refractive surgery corneal ectasia is the most dreaded complication for any refractive surgeon. Changes in biomechanical strength after refractive surgery are responsible for any such occurrence. Ocular response analyzer (ORA) measures the corneal hysteresis (CH) and the corneal resistance factor (CRF) to provide an estimate of the corneal biomechanical strength.[35,36] Both CH, which represents the ability of cornea to absorb or dampen an applied force, and CRF, which is a viscoelastic parameter, are decreased after SMILE. However, the reduction is less as compared to LASIK. The Corvis ST (Corneal Visualization Scheimpflug Technology) has also been used to document a significant reduction in the corneal biomechanical strength after SMILE.

The anatomical difference in the arrangement of collagen fibrils confers the anterior corneal stroma with the advantage of having a greater biomechanical strength when compared to the posterior stroma. SMILE has the advantage of preserving the strength of anterior stroma, which explains the increased biomechanical strength as compared to LASIK.

CONCLUSION

Small incision lenticule extraction is a safe, effective, and predictable refractive surgical procedure. It is becoming increasingly popular owing to its excellent visual outcomes and reduced risk of complications. It has the advantage of providing precise visual acuity and quality, while maintaining a stable ocular surface and the biomechanical strength of the cornea. Postoperative dry eye disease is less frequently observed after SMILE as compared to flap-based corneal ablative procedures, with a decreased dependency on artificial lubricants. At present, the use of SMILE is limited to the treatment of myopia and myopic astigmatism, with reduced predictability and stability in cases with significant astigmatism and hyperopia. Technological advancements may further expand the applications of SMILE with optimal visual and anatomical outcomes.

REFERENCES

1. Ma J, Cao NJ, Xia LK. Efficacy, safety, predictability, aberrations and corneal biomechanical parameters after SMILE and FLEx: meta-analysis. Int J Ophthalmol. 2016;9(5):757-62.
2. Sekundo W, Kunert KS, Blum M. Small incision corneal refractive surgery using the small incision lenticule extraction (SMILE) procedure for the correction of myopia and myopic astigmatism: results of a 6-month prospective study. Br J Ophthalmol. 2011;95(3):335-9.

3. Kamiya K, Shimizu K, Igarashi A, et al. Visual and refractive outcomes of small incision lenticule extraction for the correction of myopia: 1-year follow-up. BMJ Open. 2015;5(11):e008268.
4. Shah R, Shah S, Sengupta S. Results of small incision lenticule extraction: all-in-one femtosecond laser refractive surgery. J Cataract Refract Surg. 2011;37(1):127-37.
5. Zhao J, Yao P, Li M, et al. The morphology of corneal cap and its relation to refractive outcomes in femtosecond laser small incision lenticule extraction (SMILE) with anterior segment optical coherence tomography observation. PloS One. 2013;8(8):e70208.
6. Vestergaard A, Ivarsen AR, Asp S, et al. Small-incision lenticule extraction for moderate to high myopia: predictability, safety, and patient satisfaction. J Cataract Refract Surg. 2012;38(11):2003-10.
7. Lin F, Xu Y, Yang Y. Comparison of the visual results after SMILE and femtosecond laser-assisted LASIK for myopia. J Refract Surg. 2014;30(4):248-54.
8. Hjortdal JØ, Vestergaard AH, Ivarsen A, et al. Predictors for the outcome of small-incision lenticule extraction for myopia. J Refract Surg. 2012;28(12): 865-71.
9. Ganesh S, Brar S, Patel U. Comparison of ReLEx SMILE and PRK in terms of visual and refractive outcomes for the correction of low myopia. Int Ophthalmol. 2017 (Epub ahead of print).
10. Reinstein DZ, Carp GI, Archer TJ, et al. Outcomes of small incision lenticule extraction (SMILE) in low myopia. J Refract Surg. 2014;30(12):812-8.
11. Yıldırım Y, Alagöz C, Demir A, et al. Long-term results of small-incision lenticule extraction in high myopia. Turk J Ophthalmol. 2016;46(5):200-4.
12. Ivarsen A, Hjortdal J. Correction of myopic astigmatism with small incision lenticule extraction. J Refract Surg. 2014;30(4):240-7.
13. Pedersen IB, Ivarsen A, Hjortdal J. Three-year results of small incision lenticule extraction for high myopia: refractive outcomes and aberrations. J Refract Surg. 2015;31(11):719-24.
14. Wu W, Wang Y, Zhang H, et al. One-year visual outcome of small incision lenticule extraction (SMILE) surgery in high myopic eyes: retrospective cohort study. BMJ Open. 2016;6(9): e010993.
15. Liu Y-C, Teo EP, Lwin NC, et al. Early corneal wound healing and inflammatory responses after SMILE: comparison of the effects of different refractive corrections and surgical experiences. J Refract Surg. 2016;32(5):346-53.
16. Ganesh S, Brar S, Relekar KJ. Epithelial thickness profile changes following small incision refractive lenticule extraction (SMILE) for myopia and myopic astigmatism. J Refract Surg. 2016;32(7):473-82.
17. Kunert KS, Blum M, Duncker GI, et al. Surface quality of human corneal lenticules after femtosecond laser surgery for myopia comparing different laser parameters. Graefes Arch Clin Exp Ophthalmol. 2011;249(9):1417-24.
18. Blum M, Kunert K, Schröder M, et al. Femtosecond lenticule extraction for the correction of myopia: preliminary 6-month results. Graefes Arch Clin Exp Ophthalmol. 2010;248(7):1019-27.
19. Shah R, Shah S. Effect of scanning patterns on the results of femtosecond laser lenticule extraction refractive surgery. J Cataract Refract Surg. 2011; 37(9):1636-47.
20. Shetty R, Negalur N, Shroff R, et al. Cap Lenticular adhesion during small incision lenticular extraction surgery: causative factors and outcomes. Asia Pac J Ophthalmol (Phila). 2017;6(3):233-7.

21. Chen X, Wang Y, Zhang J, et al. Comparison of ocular higher-order aberrations after SMILE and Wavefront-guided Femtosecond LASIK for myopia. BMC Ophthalmol. 2017;17(1):42.
22. Sekundo W, Gertnere J, Bertelmann T, et al. One-year refractive results, contrast sensitivity, high-order aberrations and complications after myopic small-incision lenticule extraction (ReLEx SMILE). Graefes Arch Clin Exp Ophthalmol. 2014;252(5):837-43.
23. Ganesh S, Gupta R. Comparison of visual and refractive outcomes following femtosecond laser-assisted lasik with smile in patients with myopia or myopic astigmatism. J Refract Surg. 2014;30(9):590-6.
24. Agca A, Ozgurhan EB, Yildirim Y, et al. Corneal backscatter analysis by in vivo confocal microscopy: fellow eye comparison of small incision lenticule extraction and femtosecond laser-assisted LASIK. J Ophthalmol. 2014;2014:265012.
25. Dhubhghaill SN, Rozema JJ, Jongenelen S, et al. Normative values for corneal densitometry analysis by scheimpflug optical assessment corneal densitometry in the normal population. Invest Ophthalmol Vis Sci. 2014; 55(1):162-8.
26. Wang J, Simpson TL, Fonn D. Objective measurements of corneal light-backscatter during corneal swelling, by optical coherence tomography. Invest Ophthalmol Vis Sci. 2004;45(10):3493-8.
27. Sekundo W, Reinstein DZ, Blum M. Improved lenticule shape for hyperopic femtosecond lenticule extraction (ReLEx® FLEx): a pilot study. Lasers Med Sci. 2016;31(4):659-64.
28. Blum M, Kunert KS, Voßmerbäumer U, et al. Femtosecond lenticule extraction (ReLEx) for correction of hyperopia—first results. Graefes Arch Clin Exp Ophthalmol. 2013;251(1):349-55.
29. Wei S, Wang Y. Comparison of corneal sensitivity between FS-LASIK and femtosecond lenticule extraction (ReLEx flex) or small-incision lenticule extraction (ReLEx smile) for myopic eyes. Graefes Arch Clin Exp Ophthalmol. 2013;251(6):1645-54.
30. Liu M, Zhang T, Zhou Y, et al. Corneal regeneration after femtosecond laser small-incision lenticule extraction: a prospective study. Graefes Arch Clin Exp Ophthalmol. 2015;253(7):1035-42.
31. Ishii R, Shimizu K, Igarashi A, et al. Influence of femtosecond lenticule extraction and small incision lenticule extraction on corneal nerve density and ocular surface: a 1-year prospective, confocal, microscopic study. J Refract Surg. 2015;31(1):10-5.
32. Toda I. LASIK and the ocular surface. Cornea. 2008;27(Suppl 1):S70-6.
33. Chao C, Golebiowski B, Stapleton F. The role of corneal innervation in LASIK-induced neuropathic dry eye. Ocul Surf. 2014;12(1):32-45.
34. Denoyer A, Landman E, Trinh L, et al. Dry eye disease after refractive surgery: comparative outcomes of small incision lenticule extraction versus LASIK. Ophthalmology. 2015;122(4):669-76.
35. Sefat SM, Wiltfang R, Bechmann M, et al. Evaluation of changes in human corneas after femtosecond laser-assisted LASIK and small-incision lenticule extraction (SMILE) using non-contact tonometry and ultra-high-speed camera (Corvis ST). Curr Eye Res. 2016;41(7):917-22.
36. Osman IM, Helaly HA, Abdalla M, et al. Corneal biomechanical changes in eyes with small incision lenticule extraction and laser assisted in situ keratomileusis. BMC Ophthalmol. 2016;16:123.

Chapter

8

Intraoperative Complications in Small Incision Lenticule Extraction

Manpreet Kaur, Jeewan S Titiyal

INTRODUCTION

Small incision lenticule extraction (SMILE) is increasingly being preferred over flap-based corneal ablative procedures for the treatment of myopia and myopic astigmatism. Lenticule extraction through a small side-cut incision instead of raising a flap provides superior biomechanical strength and helps in the elimination of flap-related complications, such as striae, buttonholes, irregular, and dislodged flaps. Moreover, SMILE is associated with better ocular surface stability and less incidence of dry eyes.

Flap-related complications are not observed; however, SMILE is associated with unique complications related to the cap and lenticule formation that manifest during the initial learning curve (Table 8.1). A majority of complications decrease in incidence as the surgeon gains experience and becomes accustomed to the different surgical aspects of this procedure. We herein describe the etiology, predisposing factors, and management of the commonly encountered complications during SMILE along with their representative videos.

SUCTION LOSS

Incidence

The incidence of intraoperative suction loss during SMILE ranges from 0.8% to 4.4%.[1,2] The incidence may be as high as 11% for novice surgeons.[3] Suction loss may result in suboptimal visual outcomes, if it is not managed effectively (11).

Pathophysiology

The Carl Zeiss contact lens used for docking during SMILE has a curved contact surface in order to complement the corneal curvature. It is available in three different sizes [small (S), medium (M), and large (L)] based on the white-to-white diameter of different corneas. The docking is based on the principle of "acurvation" rather than applanation and the cornea is not

Table 8.1: Intraoperative complications during the initial learning curve of small incision lenticule extraction (SMILE)

Complication	Incidence	Pathophysiology	Management	Outcomes
Suction loss (11)	0.8–11%	Low-suction VisuMax system with soft docking	Protocol depending upon stage of suction loss. Redock to complete procedure or convert to excimer laser ablation (PRK/LASIK)	Satisfactory visual outcomes in majority
Black spots (12)	11–14%	Debris/air bubbles entrapped between contact lens and cornea	Clean contact lens or ocular surface	Satisfactory visual outcomes, increased adhesions during dissection
Opaque bubble layer (13)	0–51.82%	Accumulation and transient opacification of cavitation bubbles in intrastromal interface	Wait for OBL to disappear or gently massage out from interface	Delayed visual recovery with eventual satisfactory visual outcomes. Decreased scotopic contrast sensitivity Increased higher-order aberrations
Difficult lenticule extraction (14 to 17)	1.9–9%	Difficult dissection in correct plane or lenticule mis-dissection and cap-lenticular adhesions	ASOCT to identify dissection plane. Sinskey-hook-assisted dissection. Modified strippers and Y-shaped tip instruments	Delayed visual recovery. Irregular astigmatism and suboptimal visual quality. Increased likelihood of irregular interface, cap and side-cut tears, retained lenticule, epithelial defects
Retained lenticule (14 and 15)	0.6–3%	Difficult lenticule dissection or forceful extraction	Retreat: surface ablation or LASIK or circle pattern of VisuMax laser	Partially retained lenticule fragments: irregular astigmatism. Completely retained lenticule: satisfactory visual outcomes after re-treatment
Cap tears Side-cut tears (16)	0.3–16.2% 1.8–4%	Excessive surgical manipulation, forceful lenticule dissection & extraction	Frequent instillation of artificial tears. Bandage contact lens in cap tears till re-epithelialization completed	Delayed visual recovery. Satisfactory visual outcomes in majority. Cap tears may lead to stromal scarring and irregular astigmatism
Epithelial defects (17)	2–41.9%	Surgical trauma. Frequent instillation of topical anesthesia	Frequent instillation of topical artificial tears. Bandage contact lens in large defects	Satisfactory visual outcomes in majority. Central epithelial defects may induce inflammation and interface haze

(PRK: Photorefractive keratectomy; LASIK: Laser-assisted in situ keratomileusis; OBL: Opaque bubble layer; ASOCT: Anterior segment optical coherence tomography).

forced into a deformed planar, nonphysiological shape. The "soft docking" minimizes the intraocular pressure (IOP) rise as well as the tissue distortion during femtosecond laser application. It also allows the patient to maintain fixation throughout the surgical procedure. The low-pressure suction cone applies approximately 35 mm Hg pressure, which results in a maximum IOP rise of 30–80 mm Hg in various in vitro studies.[4,5] However, the low-suction system is associated with longer suction times which predisposes to intraoperative suction loss. It takes approximately 30–35 seconds for the femtosecond laser to complete the cuts (reduced to 25–28 seconds with a recent software update). Suction loss can easily occur in the presence of other predisposing factors and, if the contact lens is not properly docked.

Predisposing Factors

Various factors may contribute to an increased incidence of suction loss (Table 8.2).

Table 8.2: Predisposing factors for intraoperative suction loss and preventive measures

Predisposing factors	***Preventive measures***
Machine-related factors	
Low-suction system	Decreased total surgical time, surgeon experience
Improper vacuum tube attachment	Preoperative check of machine attachments
Contact lens size mismatch	Select contact lens as per patient's white-to-white diameter
Surgeon factors	
Improper docking	Check centration while docking, surgeon experience
Mechanical factors	
Tight speculum	Check speculum: not too tight/too loose
Improper drape	Proper draping technique
Patient factors	
Uncooperative, anxious patient	Preoperative counseling
Anatomical factors	
Narrow palpebral apertures	Proper patient positioning
Deep eye sockets	Proper patient positioning
Prominent nasal bridge	Proper patient positioning
Too dry cornea	Wet cornea with a moist merocel sponge
Excessive tearing	Dry cornea with a merocel sponge
Large cylinder power	–
Poor fixation	Patient counseling
Loose conjunctival tissue	Sweep away from center with merocel sponge, solid blade speculum
Large cap diameter	–

- *Machine-related factors*: The long suction time associated with SMILE is an inherent risk factor for suction loss which is further compounded by the surgeon inexperience. It takes around 25–35 seconds for the femtosecond laser to complete the cuts. The low-pressure VisuMax laser system also predisposes to the development of suction loss with longer duration of the procedure. Moreover, a mismatch between the contact lens and patient's white-to-white diameter increases the incidence of suction loss.
- *Surgeon factors:* Improper docking by the surgeon predisposes to suction loss. The incidence of suction loss decreases with surgeon experience; however, it cannot be totally eliminated.[6]
- *Mechanical factors:* Mechanical factors, such as a tight speculum and improper application of the surgical drape may also result in intraoperative suction loss.
- *Anatomical factors:* Eyes with narrow palpebral apertures, deep eye sockets, excessive tearing, too dry cornea, large cap diameter, large cylinder power, and poor fixation are also predisposed to develop suction loss.[2,6] Loose conjunctival tissue can interfere with successful docking and can lead to repeated suction loss.
- *Patient factors*: Patient cooperation is an essential contributory factor and an uncooperative, anxious patient that squeezes and frequently blinks the eyes during surgery has a high likelihood of experiencing suction loss.

Prevention

Preventive measures to minimize the incidence of suction loss have been summarized in Table 8.2. The machine should be calibrated preoperatively and the vacuum tube should be correctly routed. The incidence of suction loss decreases with surgeon experience and a decrease in the total duration of surgery. The contact lens should be selected according to the patient's white-to-white diameter in order to avoid any mismatch. The patient should be positioned properly and the head may be tilted slightly to avoid interference by a prominent nasal bridge. The speculum and drape should be properly applied and should not exert any undue traction. The cornea should be neither too moist nor too dry. Loose conjunctiva could be gently swept away from the central field by merocel sponges. A solid blade speculum also helps to mechanically hold the loose conjunctival tissue away from the central operative field.

Preoperative counseling is essential to calm an anxious patient and explain what is expected from the patient during laser application. The patient should be explained that the green fixation light may not be visible during femtosecond laser delivery, and the patient should not become anxious and move.

Management

Suction loss may occur during any stage of the surgical procedure, and the further management depends upon the stage at which suction loss occurs (Flowchart 8.1).[2,7] The surgeon may redock and continue the procedure, or may have to convert to laser-assisted in situ keratomileusis (LASIK) in the same sitting or at a later date. In cases where the procedure is restarted in the same sitting, the contact lens should be cleaned before redocking. Massaging the center of the cornea clears the bubble layer and provides a central reference point for recentration. Infrared light and a clear central bubble, if present, may also act as a guide during recentration. It is advisable to restart the procedure as soon as possible before the reference bubble layer disappears.

It is recommended to dock again and restart the procedure, if suction loss occurs at less than 10% posterior lenticule cut. In cases where more than 10% of posterior lenticule cut has been completed, the procedure should be converted to surface ablation or LASIK either in the same sitting or at a later date (Figs. 8.1A and B).

If suction loss occurs during lenticule side cut (posterior), it is recommended to redock and continue the procedure after decreasing the lenticule diameter by 0.2–0.4 mm. The reduced lenticule diameter ensures that the posterior limit of the lenticule is reached by the side cut over its entire length, even in the event of decentration during redocking.

The surgeon may also increase the depth of the lenticule side cut, if required, as an increased depth will ensure that the posterior limit of the lenticule is reached circumferentially in case of a change in incision depth.

Flowchart 8.1: Stepwise algorithm for management of intraoperative suction loss.

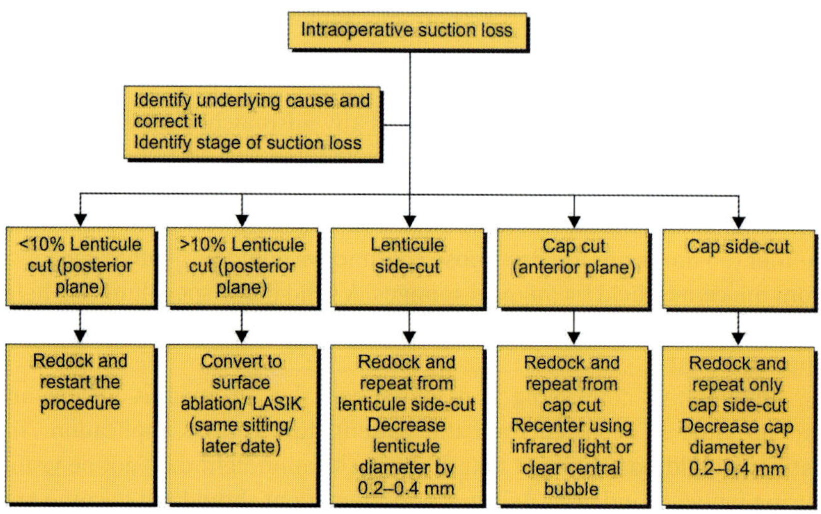

(LASIK: Laser-assisted in situ keratomileusis).

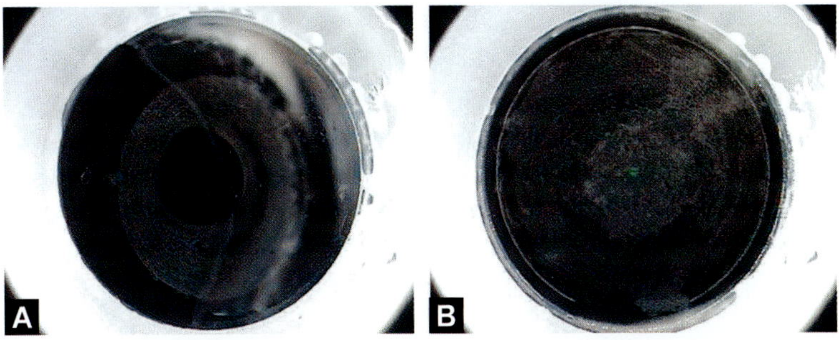

Figs. 8.1A and B: (A) Suction loss after completion of more than 10% (2.81 mm) of lenticule cut. (B) A 7.9 mm femtosecond laser flap with a superior hinge is created after redocking, in the same sitting.

Redock and continue the procedure, if suction loss occurs during cap cut (anterior plane). Centration may be achieved by using either the infrared light or the clear central bubble as a reference.

In cases with suction loss during cap side cut (anterior), only the anterior side cut needs to be created again, using the "side-cut repair module". The cap diameter is reduced by 0.2–0.4 mm in such cases. The depth of the side cut may be increased, if needed.

Outcomes

Delayed visual recovery may be present, though the final outcomes are satisfactory in a majority of cases.[2,6] Difficult lenticule extraction and monocular diplopia have been reported in a case with suction loss.[1]

It may be beneficial to avoid the second-pass procedure in the same sitting in order to minimize the possibility of an irregular interface due to the creation of two dissection planes. Repeat docking may not be possible in extensive conjunctival chemosis or hyperanxious patients. It is advisable to defer the second-pass procedure in such cases.[8]

Liu et al. evaluated the incidence and outcomes of suction loss in 8,490 eyes, and observed satisfactory visual outcomes in 35 eyes with suction loss after retreatment with femtosecond laser for incomplete SMILE.[9] The accuracy and predictability of cap thickness after double femtosecond laser pass for an incomplete SMILE cap did not significantly differ from the single pass in the fellow eyes. The patients did not perceive a difference in vision in the retreated eyes when compared with the fellow eye that underwent uneventful SMILE procedure.

We achieved optimal visual and anatomical outcomes in two cases with suction loss at varying stages of the procedure.[10] One case was converted to LASIK in the same sitting, with a larger flap diameter. The patient regained uncorrected distance visual acuity of 20/20 after the procedure. The second case experienced suction loss at the beginning of the procedure due to excessive eye movement by an anxious patient. The patient was counseled, redocked and retreated uneventfully in the same sitting.

BLACK SPOTS

Incidence

Black spots have been reported in 11–14% of cases undergoing SMILE (12).[3,10]

Mechanism

Small air bubbles or debris (glove powder, cotton fibers, mucous, etc.) may become entrapped between the applanating surface of the patient interface (PI) and the corneal surface. They may result in dark spots or black spots that are visible during femtosecond laser application (Figs. 8.2 and 8.3).

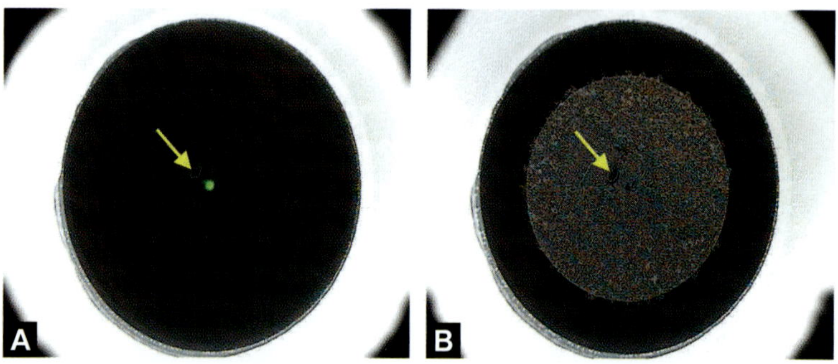

Figs. 8.2A and B: (A) Air bubble entrapped between the contact lens and ocular surface after docking (arrow: entrapped air bubble); (B) Black spot at the site of entrapped air bubble after femtosecond laser application (arrow: black spot).

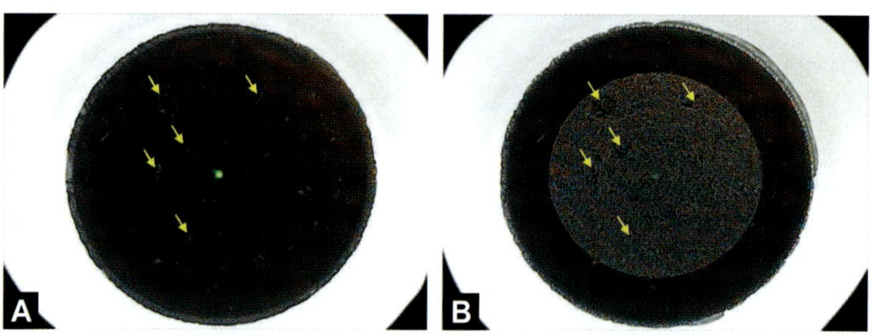

Figs. 8.3A and B: (A) Interface debris (glove powder, mucous, etc.) on the undersurface of contact lens during docking (arrows: interface debris); (B) Black spots at the site of interface debris after femtosecond laser application (arrows: black spots).

Predisposing Factors

- *Ocular surface-related factors:* Presence of debris, such as glove powder, cotton fibers, and mucous particles on the ocular surface predisposes to development of black spots.
- *Contact lens-related factors:* An unclean contact lens with debris or water droplets predisposes to black spots formation.
- *Topical anesthesia:* Frequent instillation of topical anesthesia leads to loosening of the corneal epithelium and predisposes to the development of black spots.
- *Docking-related factors:* Repeated docking attempts are associated with a higher incidence of black spots.

Clinical Significance

These black spots hamper effective femtosecond laser delivery and result in microadhesions. Difficulties may be encountered during subsequent lenticule dissection as a result of microadhesions; however, small black spots do not have an adverse effect on the visual and anatomical outcomes.[3,10]

Prevention

The incidence of black spots may be minimized by adequately wetting the cornea before docking and avoiding any debris on the ocular surface as well as the contact lens.[3] In cases with significant debris or a large air bubble observed in the interface immediately after docking, the suction should be released and the eye redocked after thoroughly irrigating the cornea as well as the applanating surface of the PI in order to remove any remnant debris. Frequent instillation of topical anesthesia should be avoided as it leads to loosening of the corneal epithelium and increases the frequency of black spots. With increasing surgeon experience, the frequency of multiple docking attempts is reduced which helps to reduce the incidence of black spots.

OPAQUE BUBBLE LAYER

Incidence

The incidence of opaque bubble layer (OBL) in SMILE is highly variable, and may range from 0% to 51.82% (13).[1,11]

Mechanism

Femtosecond laser technology is based on the principle of photodisruption, wherein the laser-induced optical breakdown (LIOB) forms plasma of free electrons and ionized molecules. Cavitation bubbles are formed by the rapid expansion of plasma and these bubbles enlarge and coalesce to form

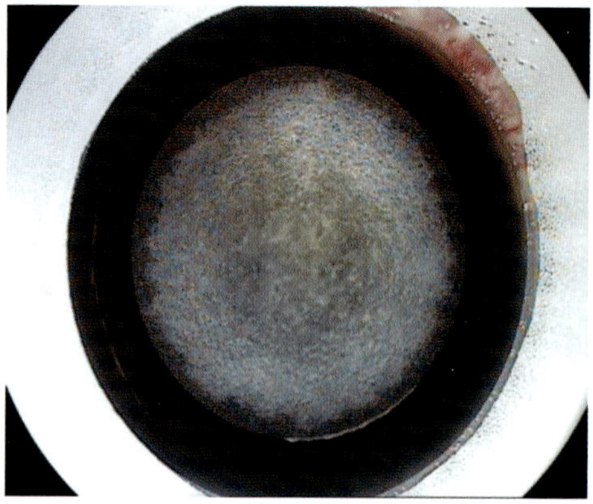

Fig. 8.4: Dense opaque bubble layer after femtosecond laser application in a case of small incision lenticule extraction (SMILE).

lamellar dissection planes in the corneal stroma. OBL is a result of the accumulation of gas bubbles temporarily entrapped in the intrastromal interface, creating transient opacity (Fig. 8.4). The corneal compression and high vacuum levels created by applanation during femtosecond laser delivery do not allow the gas bubbles to escape. The gas bubbles then infiltrate the stroma and create an opaque, whitened appearance of the cornea known as OBL. Owing to the transient nature of the phenomenon it has not been possible to describe the histopathological characteristics of OBL. However, ultra-high-resolution optical coherence tomography provides a more detailed structural analysis.[12]

Clinical Features

Two different morphological variants of OBL have been described: the early (hard) type OBL with a dense appearance that develops at the plane of laser pulses, and the late (diffuse) type OBL with a more transparent appearance that develops after the completion of laser dissection through a particular area.[13]

Predisposing Factors

- *Machine settings and laser parameters:* Machine settings and laser parameters may influence the development of OBL. Higher energy settings and increased line spacing of laser spots may lead to OBL formation. Minimal spot energy and rapid firing rate results in decreased production of bubbles and permits the femtosecond laser to remain ahead of the expanding OBL in VisuMax laser system. A decrease in spot and line spacing reduces the frequency and density of OBL.[14]
- *Surgeon factors:* It has been suggested that increased force during docking increases the risk of OBL formation. We have observed that surgeon

inexperience and repeated docking attempts increase the incidence of OBL.

- *Anatomical factors:* Other predisposing factors include eyes with thicker corneas and thinner lenticules.[11,13] Elevated corneal hysteresis is an independent predictive risk factor for OBL occurrence.[15]

Clinical Significance

The VisuMax platform is a low-vacuum system that allows the patient to maintain vision and causes a relatively lower IOP rise during treatment. However, this feature may also allow gas bubbles to travel anterior to the cap interface, potentially increasing the risk of incomplete lenticule dissection in patients with hard OBLs.[12] We observed increased incidence of tissue bridges and intralamellar adhesions during lenticule dissection in cases with OBL.[10] However, the surgery could be completed uneventfully in all cases. An excessive OBL may lead to more irregular interfaces and poorer results. In eye-tracker-based systems, the dense OBL may interfere with intraoperative tracking. It may also interfere with intraoperative pachymetry measurements because of the presence of intralamellar gas bubbles which are reflective to acoustic signals.[16]

Management

Optimal laser settings will help to minimize the incidence of OBL, and the energy settings may be customized to achieve minimal OBL with smooth lenticule formation. OBL is a transient phenomenon and the surgeon may wait for some time for the OBL to disappear. However, this may increase the intraoperative surgical duration. Alternatively, the OBL may be gently massaged out from the interface to improve visibility.

Clinical Outcomes

Overall visual outcomes are satisfactory despite OBL formation. However, mild decrease in scotopic contrast sensitivity has been observed.[17] There may be a higher incidence of flap tear and a lower predictability value.[11]

A trend toward worse visual acuity and increased higher-order aberrations has been noted in eyes with dense OBL after 3 months of surgery, with a significant increase in trefoil aberrations.[13] We observed a delayed visual recovery in our cases with OBL as a result of difficult dissection; however, the final visual outcomes were satisfactory.[10]

DIFFICULT LENTICULE EXTRACTION

Incidence

The incidence of difficult lenticule extraction ranges from 1.9% to 9%.[1,10] It is more commonly observed during the initial learning curve. We observed a

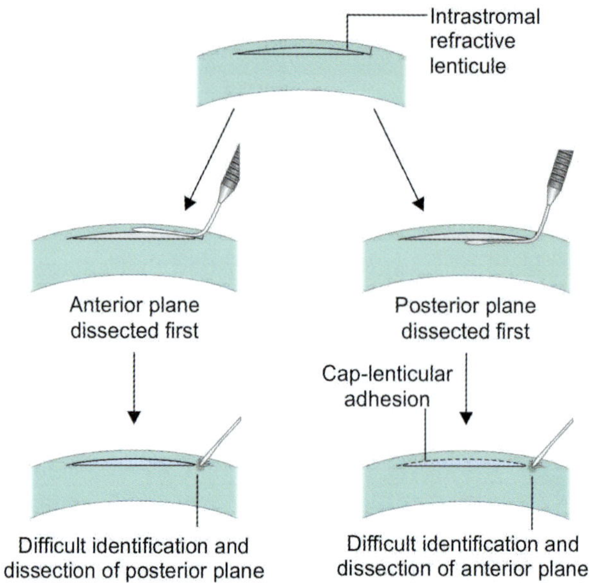

Fig. 8.5: Pathophysiology of difficult lenticule dissection and extraction.

decrease in the incidence of this complication from 16% in the initial 50 cases to 2% in the next 50 cases.[10]

Pathophysiology

Difficult lenticule extraction results from a failure to identify the correct dissection plane. Two different clinical scenarios may be observed in cases with difficult lenticule dissection, which are summarized in Figure 8.5. In the first scenario, the surgeon is in the correct dissection plane but is unable to dissect and separate the lenticule owing to increased adhesions, surgeon inexperience or difficulty in handling the thin refractive lenticules. The anterior plane is dissected first as per the described technique; however, the surgeon may not be able to identify the posterior dissection plane.

The second and most common underlying mechanism that leads to difficult lenticule dissection and extraction is an inadvertent posterior lamellar separation before completing the anterior lamellar dissection.[18,19] Ideally, the anterior lenticule plane is dissected first from the anterior cap, followed by the posterior plane. In cases where the posterior plane is dissected first, the lenticule becomes adherent to the overlying cap. The cap-lenticular adhesion makes it extremely difficult to identify the anterior dissection plane. Moreover, dissection of the anterior lenticule plane may not be possible in the absence of an adequate posterior stromal support, which is lost when the posterior plane is dissected first.

Predisposing Factors

The predisposing factors and preventive measures are summarized in Table 8.3.

- *Surgeon factors:* Surgeon inexperience is associated with difficult lenticule dissection. A novice surgeon may have difficulty in identifying the dissection plane, and may even create a false dissection plane while attempting forceful lenticule dissection. Inadvertent initial dissection of the posterior plane leads to an adherent lenticule to the anterior stromal cap. In such cases, further lenticule dissection and extraction may not be possible for novice surgeons, and the procedure may have to be abandoned.
- *Laser settings:* Optimal laser settings lead to the creation of a uniform bubble layer that facilitates smooth lenticule dissection and extraction. Too low-energy settings result in increased intralamellar tissue bridges and adhesions, thereby leading to difficulties during lamellar dissection. Too high-energy settings may result in the formation of dense OBL.
- *Opaque bubble layer:* A dense OBL may hamper smooth lenticule dissection and extraction. An increased incidence of tissue bridges and intralamellar adhesions has been observed during lenticule dissection in cases with OBL.[10]

Table 8.3: Predisposing factors and surgical tips to prevent difficult lenticule dissection

Predisposing factors	*Preventive measures*
Surgeon factors	
Surgeon inexperience	▪ Stepwise progression (observation, wetlab training, FLEx, SMILE, etc.) ▪ *Intraoperative signs*: Shimmer sign, white ring sign, etc. ▪ *Modified techniques*: Continuous curvilinear lenticulerrhexis, Chung's swing technique, modified technique with outside-in circumferential dissection
Laser settings	
Low energy: intralamellar adhesions	Optimal energy settings
High energy: opaque bubble layer	Optimal energy settings
Black spots	Clean ocular surface and contact lens
Lenticule characteristics	
Thin lenticule	Thick lenticule (high refractive error), increase minimum lenticule thickness
Low refractive error	Higher refractive error

(FLEx: Femtosecond lenticule extraction; SMILE: Small incision lenticule extraction).

- *Black spots:* Black spots result from entrapped debris or air bubble between the PI and ocular surface, and hamper femtosecond laser delivery. They result in localized microadhesions, which create difficulties during subsequent lenticule dissection.[10]
- *Lenticule characteristics:* Thin lenticules are difficult to dissect, especially during the initial training period. A positive association has been observed between decreased lenticule thickness and the incidence of cap-lenticular adhesion.[18]
- *Refractive error:* Low refractive error and manifest refraction spherical equivalent result in thinner lenticules and increased frequency of cap-lenticular adhesions.[18]

Management

Timely detection is the key to ensure optimum management in cases with difficult lenticule dissection. The management options are summarized in Flowchart 8.2. Forceful lenticule dissection should be avoided as it may lead to the creation of a false plane or lead to stromal damage.

A slit-lamp examination to confirm the lenticule dissection plane may be difficult in the presence of cap edema. An anterior segment optical coherence tomography (ASOCT) may act as an invaluable tool during difficult lenticule dissection.[20] It confirms the plane of dissection and can help to diagnose cases of cap-lenticular adhesions. A hand-held ASOCT is more useful, as it will provide an on-table assessment without the need to shift the patient to the investigative laboratory. Inability to dissect the lenticule

Flowchart 8.2: Pathophysiology and management of difficult lenticule dissection.

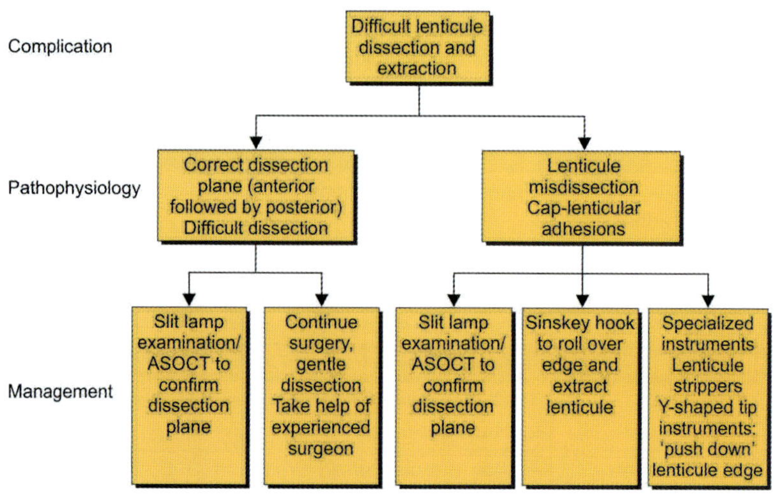

(ASOCT: Anterior segment optical coherence tomography).

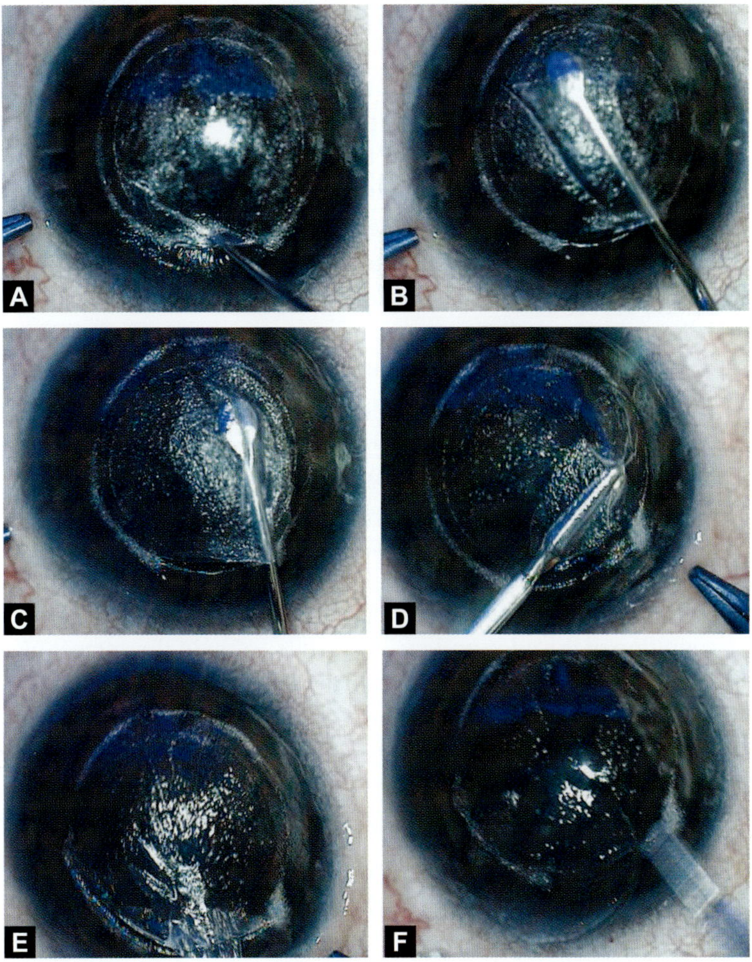

Figs. 8.6A to F: Sinskey hook-assisted lenticule extraction in a case of cap-lenticular adhesion. (A) Sinskey hook is used to nudge and evert the peripheral edge of adherent lenticule. (B and C) Blunt dissector is used to peel off the lenticule from the overlying cap by gentle sideways movements. (D and E) Forceps is used to grasp the lenticule and extract it in a circumferential manner, in order to remove any remnant adhesions. (F) Extracted lenticule is examined for its completeness.

despite being in the correct dissection plane (anterior followed by posterior) is generally associated with surgeon inexperience. After confirming that the surgeon is in the correct dissection plane, a gentle continuation of lamellar dissection may help in the completion of procedure. It is advisable to take help of a more experienced surgeon. During the initial cases, the surgeon can increase the side-cut incision width to facilitate easy lenticule extraction.

In cases with the refractive lenticule adherent to the anterior cap, a Sinskey hook may be used to facilitate lenticule extraction (Figs. 8.6A to F).[20]

The lenticule edge is gently nudged with the Sinskey hook in order to lift off a small edge of the lenticule peripherally from the anterior cap. The lenticule edge is then stripped off in a centripetal fashion till a small rolled edge of the lenticule is achieved. The separated edge can be grasped with a blunt forceps and the complete lenticule is then separated from the overlying cap by gentle sideways movement of the forceps. The separated lenticule can be successfully extracted through the side-cut incision.

It is essential to examine the extracted lenticule for its completeness, as retained lenticule fragments may lead to irregular astigmatism and sub-optimal visual outcomes.[21]

Various instruments have been devised to facilitate lenticule dissection and extraction. Customized strippers have been devised to ease lenticule extraction in cases with cap-lenticular adhesions. These instruments can be inserted into the plane between the posterior surface of lenticule and underlying stroma, and the lenticule is then directly hooked out.[19]

The identification of the lenticule edge may be particularly challenging for beginners. Instruments with a Y-shaped tip have been developed to push up the lenticule edge from the stromal bed prior to dissection.[22] This enables easy recognition of the edge and facilitates dissection in the correct plane. A "push-down" technique with the Y-shaped instruments has been described in cases with cap-lenticular adhesions.[22] The instrument is used to engage the edge of the lenticule and push it down to make room to introduce the dissector, followed by dissection of the lenticule from the cap using the dissector.

In cases with partially or completely retained lenticule, retreatment will have to be planned at a later date. A time period of at least 3 months should be allowed to elapse before attempting retreatment, in order to allow time for refractive stabilization. It is essential to repeat the preoperative workup, including cycloplegic and manifest refraction.

Partially retained lenticule fragments may lead to irregular astigmatism and may be challenging to treat.[21] Topography-guided photorefractive keratectomy has been tried; however, postoperative haze may limit the visual outcomes.[23]

The various surgical options for retreatment in cases with completely retained lenticule include surface ablation, flap-based excimer laser ablation, and circle pattern of VisuMax laser. The retreatment options have been described in detail in Chapter 10.

Prevention

The surgical tips to minimize difficult lenticule dissection and facilitate a smooth surgery are summarized in Table 8.3. It is advisable to select cases with high refractive error during the initial training period, as low refractive error with resultant thin lenticules may be difficult to handle. The minimum lenticule thickness should be increased in cases with low refractive errors. Stepwise progression from initial observation, followed by wetlab training and femtosecond lenticule extraction (FLEx) before attempting SMILE may help the surgeon to become accustomed to lenticule dissection and separation. Optimal laser settings and a clean contact lens minimize the incidence of OBL, intralamellar adhesions, and black spots.

Intraoperative signs, such as the "white-ring sign" and "shimmer sign" have been described to identify the correct dissection plane.[18,24] Various surgical techniques have been described to facilitate lenticule dissection and extraction.

Zhao et al. recommend tearing and extracting the lenticule from the stromal bed in a continuous circumferential manner without performing lamellar dissection and separation of the lenticule from the surrounding stroma.[25] The "continuous curvilinear lenticulerrhexis (CCL)" technique was observed to be safe and effective even during the learning curve and reduced the disturbance to the corneal tissue by instruments. However, it may lead to ripping of the lenticule and retained lenticule fragments, especially in cases with low myopia and resultant thin lenticules. This may lead to prolonged surgical times and repeated attempts. Moreover, this technique is contraindicated in cases with OBL formation or uneven laser scanning, thereby limiting its widespread usage. The lenticule edge needs to be identified and separated before grasping it with forceps, which may be difficult in the initial cases.

Kim et al. described "Chung's swing technique", wherein the posterior lenticule plane is separated first with a fan-shaped spatula.[26] Once the posterior interface is separated, the anterior interface of the lenticule is identified by lifting and swinging the spatula tip at the left end of the incision and is separated into a fan shape. The lenticule is grasped with a McPherson forceps at 12 o'clock, pushed toward the center of the cornea and pulled, in order to remove the lenticule in a clockwise direction. The lenticule is not separated at the 12 o'clock to 3 o'clock and the 8 o'clock to 11 o'clock positions in order to avoid damage by forceps during lenticule extraction. This may potentially increase the risk of remnant lenticule fragments, though the authors did not report such adverse effects. Lower operation times were reported with this technique; however, it was associated with increased incidence of incisional edge tearing.

Jacob et al. have also recommended creating two lamellar channels in opposite directions anterior and posterior to the lenticule in cases with thin lenticules.[27] Anterior lamellar dissection is done first, followed by central posterior lamellar dissection. A thin peripheral rim is left undissected along with the lenticule side cut. A sequential segmental dissection of the lenticule side cut is then undertaken in a manner that fixates the lenticule and allows a smooth and complete dissection of the posterior lamellar cut.

We prefer a modified technique to ensure easy identification of the correct plane of dissection. After successful femtosecond laser delivery, a double ring is observed as a result of disparity between the anterior cap and the posterior lenticule diameter. The side-cut is opened, and a lamellar dissector is introduced through the left side of the incision (for a right-handed surgeon), taking care to remain in the area between the two rings. A small circumferential strip is dissected. This step ensures that the instrument is in the correct anterior dissection plane. The dissector is then introduced in the posterior plane at 12 o'clock position, and advanced with minimal sideways movements toward the right-hand side (for the right-handed surgeon), till an adequate posterior separation of the lenticule edge is achieved. After separating the edge, the anterior plane is dissected completely till the outer margin of the double ring. The dissection progresses from left to right through the initially dissected circumferential strip. "Outside-in" movements that reach up to the outer margin of the double ring confirm the correct dissection plane. This is followed by posterior plane dissection through the pocket created initially in the right side. The separated lenticule can be easily extracted with the dissector by circumferential motions, without the need to use a forceps to grasp the lenticule.

Clinical Significance and Outcomes

Difficult lenticule extraction may result in a myriad of potential complications (Fig. 8.7 and 14 to 17).[10] Excessive surgical manipulation in such cases may lead to stromal irregularities and an irregular interface (Figs. 8.8A and B). Bowman membrane microdistortions may be observed.[18] Epithelial abrasions may occur at the site of side cut (Fig. 8.9). Side cut extension, side cut tears, and cap tears may occur (Figs. 8.10 and 8.11). Moreover, forceful lenticule extraction before completing the dissection of anterior as well as

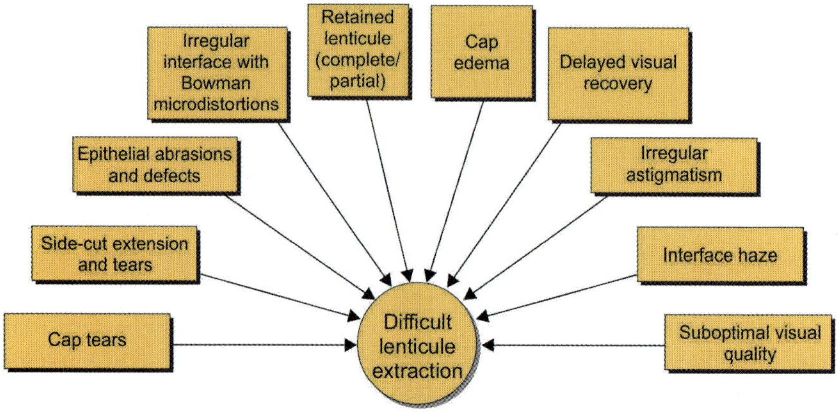

Fig. 8.7: Adverse anatomical and physiological effects of difficult lenticule extraction.

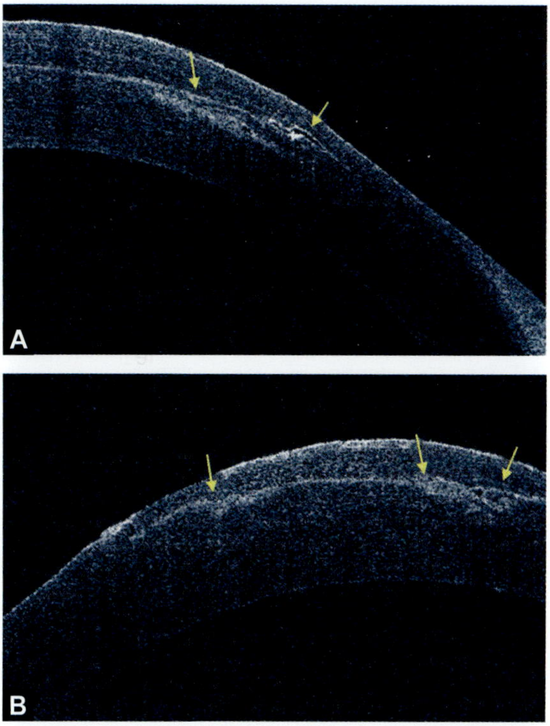

Figs. 8.8A and B: Posterior stromal damage in a case of difficult lenticule dissection as observed on anterior segment optical coherence tomography (ASOCT) (arrows: site of posterior stromal damage).

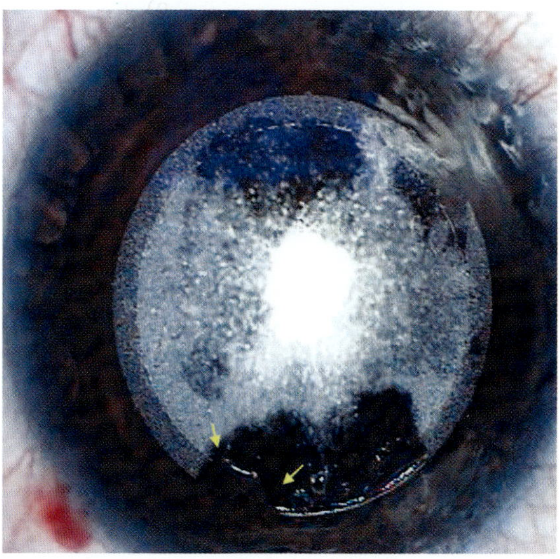

Fig. 8.9: Localized epithelial defect at the site of side cut in a case of small incision lenticule extraction (SMILE) (arrows: extent of epithelial defect).

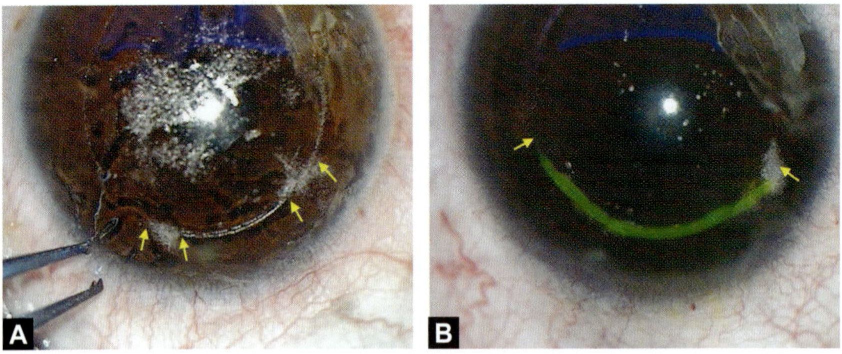

Figs. 8.10A and B: Side-cut extension in a case with excessive surgical manipulation (arrows: extent of side-cut extension); (B) Side-cut tear in a case of difficult lenticule dissection with overlying localized epithelial defect (arrows: extent of side-cut tear).

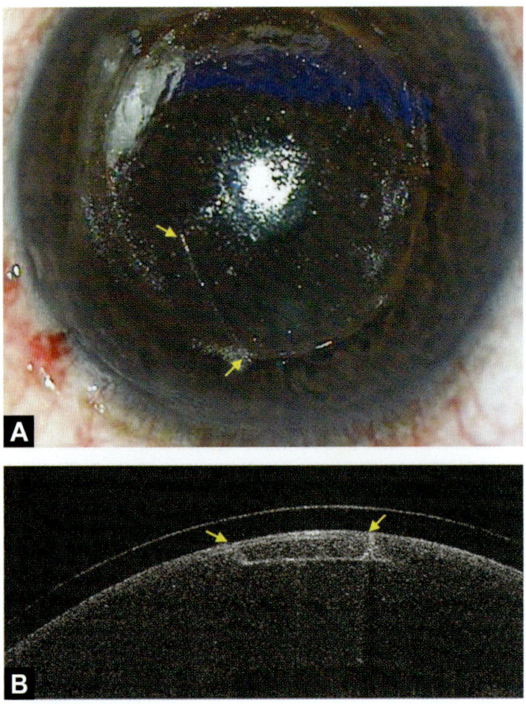

Figs. 8.11A and B: (A) Paracentral cap tear in a case of difficult lenticule extraction (arrows: extent of cap tear); (B) Superficial stromal scarring observed after 1 week in a case of cap tear. Bandage contact lens is in situ (arrows: extent of cap tear).

posterior lenticule plane may result in remnant lenticule fragments with resultant irregular astigmatism (Figs. 8.12A and B).[21] It may not be possible to successfully dissect and extract the lenticule, leading to a completely retained lenticule (Fig. 8.13).[10]

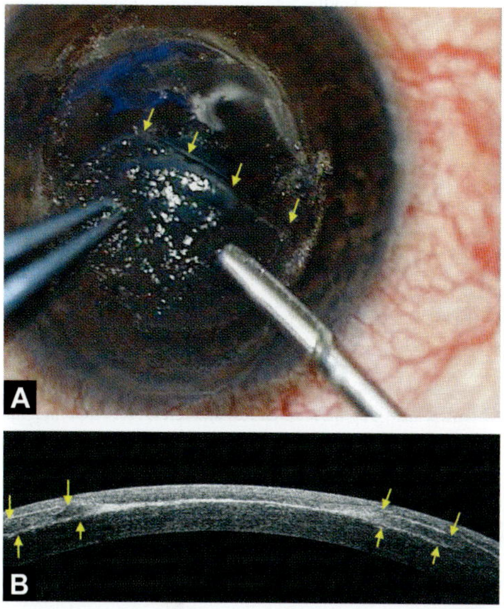

Figs. 8.12A and B: (A) Incomplete extracted lenticule with partially retained fragments in a case of difficult lenticule extraction (arrows: torn edge of extracted lenticule); (B) Retained lenticule fragments observed on anterior segment optical coherence tomography (ASOCT) (arrows: partially retained lenticule fragments).

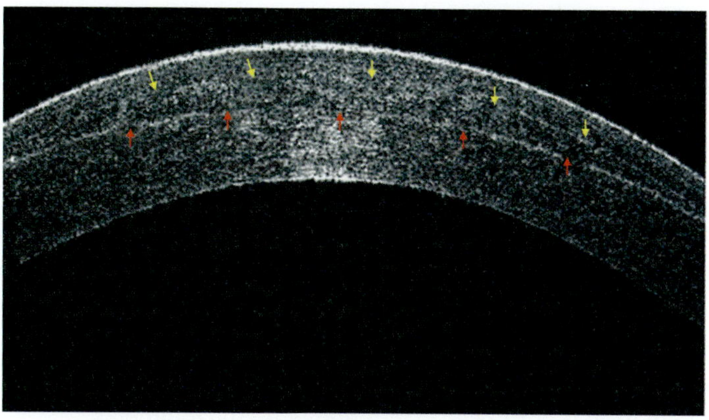

Fig. 8.13: Completely retained small incision lenticule extraction (SMILE) lenticule in a case of cap-lenticular adhesion as observed on anterior segment optical coherence tomography (ASOCT) (yellow arrows: anterior dissection plane with cap-lenticular adhesion, red arrows: posterior dissection plane).

Incorrect identification of the plane of dissection increases tissue handling and total surgical time. A delayed visual recovery is present, and suboptimal visual quality may be observed in the postoperative period as evidenced by the lower values of modulation transfer function and Strehl ratio.[18] Cap edema and interface haze are often transient and resolve with time. An irregular interface with haze may persist in cases with excessive surgical manipulation.

We observed delayed visual recovery in our cases with difficult lenticule dissection.[10] The eventual visual outcomes were satisfactory in a majority of patients; however, suboptimal visual outcomes persisted in cases with coexistent complications, such as cap tears or partially retained lenticule fragments.

RETAINED LENTICULE

Incidence

Retained lenticule is a relatively rare complication, with an incidence of 0.6–3% (14 and 15).[1,10]

Predisposing Factors

- *Laser settings*: Optimal energy settings are a prerequisite for proper lenticule creation. Inadequate laser energy settings may not lead to the formation of a uniform cavitation bubble layer. Improper lenticule creation and residual adhesions will not allow effective lenticule dissection and extraction, leading to high incidence of retained lenticule.
- *Surgeon factors*: Surgeon inexperience is associated with an increased incidence of retained lenticule. It may be particularly challenging to identify the lenticule edge as well as the correct dissection plane during the initial cases.

  Improper surgical technique may also be responsible for retained lenticule fragments or completely retained lenticule. Lenticule misdissection, wherein the posterior plane is dissected first before the anterior plane resulting in cap-lenticular adhesions predisposes to the retention of lenticule fragments. Moreover, attempting forceful lenticule extraction before separating the lenticule from the adjacent stroma may result in lenticule tear with retained fragments.
- *Opaque bubble layer*: OBL is a risk factor for difficult lenticule dissection, which in itself predisposes to retained lenticule fragments.
- *Black spots*: Extensive black spots result in microadhesions due to ineffective femtosecond laser delivery. The resultant difficulties faced during lenticule dissection and extraction may lead to retained lenticule fragments.

Prevention

Optimal laser energy settings should be used to ensure proper lenticule formation. Surgeons in the initial training period should seek help from an experienced surgeon when experiencing difficulties in lenticule dissection. Forceful lenticule extraction should be avoided to prevent tearing of the lenticule and retained fragments. An intraoperative ASOCT may be useful in cases with difficult lenticule dissection.[20]

Management and Clinical Outcomes

After extracting the SMILE lenticule, it should be carefully examined for its completeness in order to detect any partially retained fragments. If partially retained lenticule fragments are identified on-table, an attempt may be made to remove them with a blunt forceps. However, it may not be feasible to successfully extract the retained lenticule fragments in cases with significant cap edema as a result of excessive surgical manipulations. Partially retained lenticule fragments may result in irregular astigmatism and suboptimal visual outcomes (*see* Figs. 8.12A and B).[10] Cases with small peripheral fragments may be observed, as the visual outcomes may be satisfactory after postoperative corneal remodeling. Customized surface ablation may be attempted; however, the visual outcomes may be limited by the development of postoperative haze.[23]

Completely retained lenticules may be retreated at a later date with surface or flap-based excimer laser ablation, or the circle pattern of VisuMax laser, as described in Chapter 10 "Post-SMILE Enhancement and Retreatment" (*see* Fig. 8.13). It is essential to repeat the refractive workup before performing retreatment and allow a time period of 3 months to elapse before the second procedure. Satisfactory visual outcomes can be achieved in these cases.[1,10]

We have observed satisfactory visual outcomes in all cases with completely retained lenticule after retreating with LASIK. Partially retained lenticule fragments and the resultant irregular astigmatism are more challenging to manage, and optimal visual quality may not be achieved in these cases.

CAP AND SIDE-CUT TEARS

Incidence

The incidence of cap tears range from 0.3% to as high as 16.2%.[1,3,10] Side-cut extension and tears may be observed in 1.8–4% cases (16).[1,10]

Predisposing Factors

Side-cut tears and cap tears are associated with excessive surgical manipulations which may be observed in novice surgeons or during difficult lenticule dissection. Small incision size of the side cut and sudden patient movements during lenticule dissection or extraction predispose to the development of side cut or cap tears (*see* Figs. 8.10 and 8.11). Forceful extraction of lenticule without proper dissection may lead to rupture of the overlying cap and tear of the side-cut incision. Bulky surgical instruments such as forceps may entangle at the site of the side cut and result in its tear.

Prevention

Forceful lenticule dissection and extraction should be avoided. The instruments should be nonbulky, and their hub should not entangle at the site of side cut during lamellar dissection.

Management

Side-cut tears do not require any additional intervention and may be observed till the overlying epithelial abrasions are resolved. A bandage contact lens should be applied in cases with cap tear till epithelial healing is complete.

Outcomes

The visual outcomes after side-cut tears are satisfactory, though an initial delayed visual recovery may be present. The delayed visual recovery may be attributed to the coexistent cap edema due to excessive surgical manipulation, rather than as a result of side-cut tear.

Radial cap tears may result in irregular astigmatism; especially, if they encroach the visual axis.[10] Superficial scarring may be observed after healing. Peripheral cap tears may not significantly affect the visual outcomes.

EPITHELIAL DEFECTS

Incidence

Epithelial defects and minor abrasions are one of the most ubiquitous complications, with an incidence ranging from 2% to as high as 41.9% (17).[1,3,10]

Predisposing Factors

Epithelial defects and abrasions result from inadvertent epithelial trauma during surgery. Surgeon inexperience, prolonged duration of surgery, and excessive surgical manipulations predispose to the development of epithelial defects. Preoperative frequent instillation of topical anesthesia may lead to loosening of corneal epithelium and result in epithelial defects. They are more frequently observed at the site of anterior side cut, owing to repeated manipulation during the entry of instruments (*see* Fig. 8.9).

Management

Peripheral small abrasions at the site of side cut do not need any specific intervention and may be observed. Frequent instillation of artificial tears alleviates the patient's discomfort and promotes re-epithelialization.

A bandage contact lens may be applied in cases with a large central epithelial defect till completion of epithelialization. Frequent instillation of artificial tears is also recommended.

Clinical Outcomes

Small epithelial defects do not have a significant effect on the visual outcomes, though delayed visual recovery may be present.[10] Central epithelial defects may incite interface inflammation and haze.[1]

CONCLUSION

The flap-to-cap transition in SMILE is associated with intraoperative complications that are unique to the surgical procedure. The initial cases are more challenging for the surgeon, and we observed a higher incidence of complications in our initial 50 cases. The frequency decreases with surgeon experience; however, they are not completely eliminated. Optimal laser settings and following proper surgical technique can help to minimize the incidence of complications. Satisfactory visual and anatomical outcomes can be achieved in a majority of cases, though delayed visual recovery may be observed.

REFERENCES

1. Ivarsen A, Asp S, Hjortdal J. Safety and complications of more than 1500 small-incision lenticule extraction procedures. Ophthalmology. 2014;121(4):822-8.
2. Wong CW, Chan C, Tan D, et al. Incidence and management of suction loss in refractive lenticule extraction. J Cataract Refract Surg. 2014;40(12):2002-10.
3. Ramirez-Miranda A, Ramirez-Luquin T, Navas A, et al. Refractive lenticule extraction complications. Cornea. 2015;34(Suppl 10):S65-7.
4. Vetter JM, Faust M, Gericke A, et al. Intraocular pressure measurements during flap preparation using 2 femtosecond lasers and 1 microkeratome in human donor eyes. J Cataract Refract Surg. 2012;38(11):2011-8.
5. Ang M, Chaurasia SS, Angunawela RI, et al. Femtosecond lenticule extraction (FLEx): clinical results, interface evaluation, and intraocular pressure variation. Invest Ophthalmol Vis Sci. 2012;53(3):1414-21.
6. Osman IM, Awad R, Shi W, et al. Suction loss during femtosecond laser-assisted small-incision lenticule extraction: Incidence and analysis of risk factors. J Cataract Refract Surg. 2016;42(2):246-50.
7. Carl Zeiss Meditec AG. FLEx Option. Germany, Jena: Visante Operation Manual; 2011. pp. 24-5.
8. Smadja D, Santhiago MR, Mello GR, et al. Suction loss during thin-flap Femto-LASIK: management and beneficial refractive effect of the epithelium. J Cataract Refract Surg. 2012;38(5):902-5.
9. Liu M, Wang J, Zhong W, et al. Impact of suction loss during small incision lenticule extraction (SMILE). J Refract Surg. 2016;32(10):686-92.
10. Titiyal JS, Kaur M, Rathi A, et al. Learning curve of small incision lenticule extraction: challenges & complications. Cornea. 2017 Aug 9. [Epub ahead of print]
11. Son G, Lee J, Jang C, et al. Possible Risk Factors and Clinical Effects of Opaque Bubble Layer in Small Incision Lenticule Extraction (SMILE). J Refract Surg. 2017;33(1):24-9.
12. Hurmeric V, Yoo SH, Fishler J, et al. In vivo structural characteristics of the femtosecond LASIK-induced opaque bubble layers with ultrahigh-resolution SD-OCT. Ophthalmic Surg Lasers Imaging. 2010;41(Suppl):S109-13.

13. Kaiserman I, Maresky HS, Bahar I, et al. Incidence, possible risk factors, and potential effects of an opaque bubble layer created by a femtosecond laser. J Cataract Refract Surg. 2008;34(3):417-23.
14. Kanellopoulos AJ, Asimellis G. Essential opaque bubble layer elimination with novel LASIK flap settings in the FS200 Femtosecond Laser. Clin Ophthalmol. 2013;7:765-70.
15. Courtin R, Saad A, Guilbert E, et al. Opaque bubble layer risk factors in femtosecond laser-assisted LASIK. J Refract Surg. 2015;31(9):608-12.
16. Luengo Gimeno F, Chan CM, Li L, et al. Comparison of eye-tracking success in laser in situ keratomileusis after flap creation with 2 femtosecond laser models. J Cataract Refract Surg. 2011;37(3):538-43.
17. Liu CH, Sun CC, Hui-Kang Ma D, et al. Opaque bubble layer: incidence, risk factors, and clinical relevance. J Cataract Refract Surg. 2014;40(3):435-40.
18. Shetty R, Negalur N, Shroff R, et al. Cap lenticular adhesion during small incision lenticular extraction surgery: causative factors and outcomes. Asia Pac J Ophthalmol (Phila). 2017;6(3):233-7.
19. Liu YC, Pujara T, Mehta JS. New instruments for lenticule extraction in small incision lenticule extraction (SMILE). PLoS One. 2014;9(12):e113774.
20. Titiyal JS, Rathi A, Kaur M, et al. AS-OCT as a rescue tool during difficult lenticule extraction in SMILE. J Refract Surg. 2017;33(5):352-4.
21. Dong Z, Zhou X. Irregular astigmatism after femtosecond laser refractive lenticule extraction. J Cataract Refract Surg. 2013;39(6):952-4.
22. Hamed A, Fekry A. Refractive small-incision lenticule extraction: push-up and push-down techniques. J Cataract Refract Surg. 2016;42(12):1713-5.
23. Ivarsen A, Hjortdal JØ. Topography-guided photorefractive keratectomy for irregular astigmatism after small incision lenticule extraction. J Refract Surg. 2014;30(6):429-32.
24. Jacob S, Nariani A, Figus M, et al. White ring sign for uneventful lenticule separation in small-incision lenticule extraction. J Cataract Refract Surg. 2016;42(9):1251-4.
25. Zhao Y, Li M, Yao P, et al. Development of the continuous curvilinear lenticulerrhexis technique for small incision lenticule extraction. J Refract Surg. 2015;31(1):16-21.
26. Kim BK, Mun SJ, Lee DG, et al. Chung's swing technique: a new technique for small-incision lenticule extraction. BMC Ophthalmol. 2016;16(1):154.
27. Jacob S, Agarwal A, Mazzotta C, et al. Sequential segmental terminal lenticular side-cut dissection for safe and effective small-incision lenticule extraction in thin lenticules. J Cataract Refract Surg. 2017;43(4):443-8.

Chapter

9

Postoperative Complications in Small Incision Lenticule Extraction

Ruchita Falera, Manpreet Kaur, Anand Singh Brar, Jeewan S Titiyal

INTRODUCTION

Small incision lenticule extraction (SMILE) is a new refractive surgical procedure which has been approved for the correction of myopia and myopic astigmatism. It involves the creation of an intrastromal lenticule which is mechanically dissected from the surrounding stroma and removed via a 2–5 mm arcuate side cut.

The efficacy, safety, and predictability of SMILE are comparable to femtosecond laser-assisted in situ keratomileusis (LASIK). However, difficulties may be experienced during the procedure as well as in the postoperative period (Table 9.1).

The postoperative complications in SMILE may range from self-limiting transient interface haze and cap edema to potentially sight threatening corneal ectasia and infectious keratitis. The overall incidence of postoperative complications is approximately 10.8%.[1]

In this chapter, we describe the incidence, predisposing factors, management, and outcomes of the postoperative complications observed after SMILE.

INTERFACE HAZE

Incidence

Interface haze is one of the most frequent complications observed in patients undergoing SMILE, with an incidence ranging from 5.4% to as high as 54% (Figs. 9.1A to C).[1,2]

Pathophysiology

Postoperative inflammation significantly influences the process of corneal wound healing and is closely associated with interface haze. Experimental animal studies have observed scarce inflammatory cells and less deposition of extracellular matrix in corneas treated with SMILE as compared to femtosecond LASIK; thereby resulting in less interface haze.[3,4] This is attributed to an increased energy absorption from the excimer laser in patients undergoing LASIK.

Table 9.1: Incidence, risk factors, preventive measures, management and outcomes of postoperative complications after small incision lenticule extraction (SMILE)

Complication	*Incidence*	*Predisposing factors*	*Prevention*	*Management*	*Outcome*
Interface haze	5.4–54%	▪ Inexperienced surgeon ▪ Higher pulse energy ▪ Epithelial ingrowth ▪ Retreatment	▪ Optimized laser energy ▪ Use of MMC with PRK in retreatment	▪ Spontaneous resolution ▪ Increased topical steroids	▪ Self-limiting ▪ Visual outcomes satisfactory
Dry eye	3.2–32%	▪ Preexisting dry eye disease	Avoid patient with preexisting mild dry eye	▪ Frequent lubrication ▪ Anti-inflammatory drugs, cyclosporine A	▪ Self-limiting ▪ Visual outcomes satisfactory
Cap microstriae	0.4–15.4%	▪ Older patients ▪ High refractive error	Gentle cap massage after lenticule extraction	▪ Gentle cap massage ▪ Frequent topical steroids	▪ Self-limiting ▪ Visual outcomes satisfactory
Epithelial ingrowth	0.5–0.66%	▪ Epithelial defect ▪ Anterior basement membrane dystrophy ▪ Inexperienced surgeon ▪ Old age, diabetes mellitus ▪ Enhancement procedures	▪ Avoid excessive intraoperative manipulation ▪ Avoid interface handling	▪ Observation ▪ Scraping off the epithelial cells ▪ Conversion into flap and scraping off the epithelial cells ▪ Suturing of flap/use of fibrin adhesive	▪ Visual outcomes satisfactory in mild cases ▪ Irregular astigmatism, loss of BCVA in severe cases
Undercorrections, overcorrections, and postoperative regression	2.1–4% require enhancement	▪ Age >35 years ▪ Myopia >6 D ▪ Astigmatism >3 D ▪ Machine nomogram ▪ Suction loss ▪ Inexperienced surgeon	Careful patient selection	Enhancement procedures ▪ PRK with MMC ▪ Secondary LASIK ▪ Circle pattern of VisuMax laser ▪ Sub-cap-lenticule extraction	▪ Satisfactory visual outcomes ▪ Postoperative haze may limit visual recovery after PRK
Irregular topography	0.5–1%	▪ Increased intraoperative manipulation	Avoid rough dissection and forceful lenticule extraction	▪ Observation ▪ Topography-guided PRK	▪ Good outcomes with topography-guided PRK + MMC

Contd…

Contd…

Complication	Incidence	Predisposing factors	Prevention	Management	Outcome
		▪ OBL ▪ Lower spot energy with closer spots ▪ Inexperienced surgeon			
Optical aberrations	0.2–0.4%	▪ Excessive intraoperative manipulation ▪ Retained lenticule ▪ Decentered treatment ▪ Epithelial ingrowth	Avoid rough dissection and forceful lenticule extraction	▪ Observation ▪ Topography-guided PRK ▪ Enhancement procedures	▪ Good outcomes with topography-guided PRK
Decentered treatment	90% within 0.3 mm of the visual axis	▪ Large angle kappa ▪ Inexperienced surgeon	Careful centration during application of suction	▪ Observation ▪ Topography-guided PRK	▪ Good visual outcomes with PRK + MMC
Ectasia	2 case reports	▪ Keratoconus ▪ Low RSBT ▪ High refractive error ▪ Preoperative topographic abnormalities	Careful selection of patients	▪ CXL + SMILE ▪ ICRS + CXL	▪ ICRS + CXL may help to achieve optimal outcomes
Diffuse lamellar keratitis	1.6%	▪ Interface debris ▪ Thin lenticule ▪ Large lenticule diameter ▪ Surgeon inexperience ▪ High pulse energy	▪ Thorough interface irrigation at end of surgery ▪ Optimal laser energy settings ▪ Smooth tissue handling	▪ Mild cases: Frequent topical steroids ▪ Severe cases: Interface irrigation, topical and oral steroids	▪ Good visual and anatomical outcomes ▪ Majority resolve in 1–2 weeks
Infective keratitis	0.3%	▪ Surgeons' hands ▪ Contaminated surgical instruments ▪ Environmental factors ▪ Periocular flora	Surgical asepsis	▪ Irrigation of stromal pocket ▪ Topical concentrated antibiotics ▪ Cap amputation ▪ Therapeutic PK	▪ Good visual outcomes and resolution of infiltrates with empirical antibiotic treatment

(MMC: Mitomycin C; PRK: Photorefractive keratectomy; BCVA: Best corrected visual acuity; LASIK: Laser-assisted in situ keratomileusis; OBL: Opaque bubble layer; RSBT: Residual stromal bed thickness; CXL: Collagen crosslinking; ICRS: Intrastromal corneal ring segments; PK: Penetrating keratoplasty).

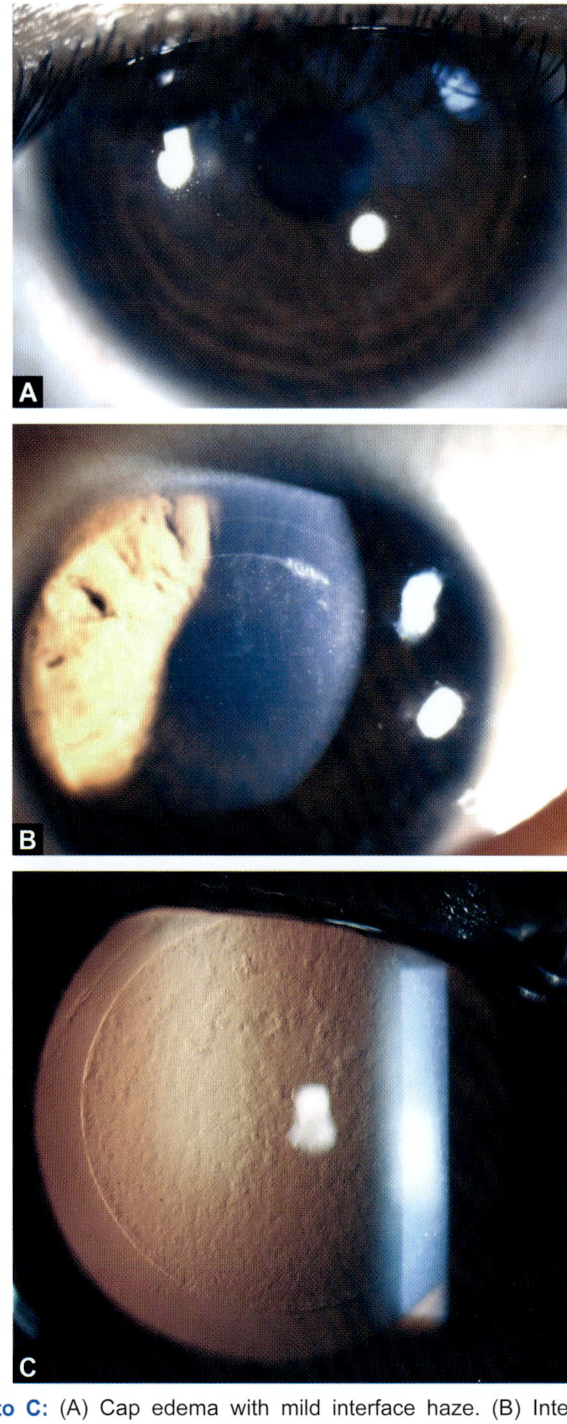

Figs. 9.1A to C: (A) Cap edema with mild interface haze. (B) Interface haze on postoperative day 1 in a case with excessive surgical manipulation during SMILE. (C) Persistent interface haze after 3 months in a case with difficult lenticule dissection.

Confocal microscopy of the SMILE interface by Agca et al. revealed a significant increase in postoperative values of interface backscatter in SMILE-treated eyes.[5] The increased backscatter persisted for up to 3 months postoperatively, which may explain the delayed visual recovery in these patients. However, no significant long-term difference in visual outcomes was observed.

The increased haze in the early postoperative period may be attributed to the increased manipulation during the dissection and extraction of the lenticule in SMILE. Suboptimal cutting of the stromal fibers by the femtosecond laser may also explain the postoperative interface scatter and haze.

Predisposing Factors

- *Surgeon factors*: Excessive intraoperative manipulation during lenticule separation, difficult lenticule extraction, and long duration of surgery may result in increased inflammation and subsequent haze.
- *Laser settings*: Use of higher pulse energy during treatment can result in greater postoperative interface haze.
- *Epithelial ingrowth:* Epithelial ingrowth in the stromal interface may lead to interface haze and hence suboptimal visual gain.
- *Retreatment*: Retreatment done in the form of photorefractive keratectomy (PRK) or LASIK can predispose to the development of interface haze. Multiple refractive procedures lead to disturbances in the stromal lamellae and can cause the haze to be more persistent.

Prevention

Optimizing laser energy, spot size, and spacing could potentially create a more "smooth" stromal cut and minimize the delayed visual recovery. Mitomycin C (MMC) should be used in cases undergoing retreatment with PRK to prevent the development of persistent interface haze.[1] Smooth surgical dissection with minimal manipulation also minimizes the incidence of interface haze.

Management

Interface haze seen after SMILE is usually transient in nature and disappears within 1 week. Resolution is spontaneous and generally does not require treatment. An increased frequency of topical steroids in the early postoperative period may help minimize inflammation and hasten the resolution of interface haze.

Outcomes

Visual outcomes are usually satisfactory, as the haze is self-limiting in nature. Persistent haze after retreatment may result in suboptimal outcomes.[1]

DRY EYE

Incidence

Postoperative dry eyes may be commonly observed after SMILE and the incidence ranges from 3.2% to 32%.[1,2] The incidence and severity is less than flap-based corneal ablative procedures.[2]

Pathophysiology

The transection of the sub-basal nerve plexus at the site of side-cut incision results in reduced corneal sensitivity and leads to postoperative dry eyes.

In the absence of the flap and a small size of the incision, there is a decreased likelihood of cutting corneal nerves and hence less postoperative dry eyes as compared to LASIK. Studies suggest less severe denervation and accelerated neuronal healing with SMILE than with LASIK.[6,7] The decreased inflammation in the postoperative period due to lesser laser energy exposure in these patients may also account for the decrease in dry eye symptoms. More severe dry eyes may be seen in patients with pre-existing compromised ocular surface or those with history of contact lens.

Prevention

A preoperative comprehensive workup is essential to rule out pre-existing compromised ocular surface and dry eyes before undertaking any refractive procedure. History regarding use of contact lens, pre-existing dry eyes, and autoimmune disease should be elicited. Ocular surface examination like fluorescein staining, Schirmer's test, and tear-film breakup time (TBUT) should be done in all patients to look for dry eye conditions.

Management

Frequent instillation of lubricants may be required in these patients. In cases where the symptoms persist, topical anti-inflammatory drugs like cyclosporine A (0.05%) may provide symptomatic relief. Patients with severe dry eyes should be dissuaded for refractive surgery.

Outcomes

Mild dry eyes are frequently observed in the early postoperative period after SMILE, which improve over time and do not affect the visual outcome.

CAP MICROSTRIAE

Incidence

The incidence of microstriae after SMILE ranges from 0.4% to 15.7%.[2,8]

Pathophysiology

Microstriae are fine hair-like irregularities in the Bowman's layer. SMILE involves the extraction of an intrastromal refractive lenticule via a small side incision. This alters the original cap-stromal bed relationship, and the redundant cap tissue in the optical zone may manifest as microstriae when the cap is not properly apposed to the stromal bed.

Predisposing Factors

- *Age of patient*: Older patients are at a greater risk of developing microstriae. Age-related increased stiffness of the cornea prevents easy recoil of the cap on the stromal bed thereby causing microstriae.
- *Refractive error*: Correction of higher refractive errors would necessitate greater amount of stromal tissue to be removed. This would alter the relation between the cap and the stromal bed, thus causing microstriae.

Management

Microstriae may be prevented by massaging the cap in a centrifugal fashion with a moist sponge after extracting the lenticule. This will ensure even distribution of the cap over the residual stromal bed. Frequent instillation of topical steroids in the early postoperative period may be beneficial.

Outcomes

In most cases, cap microstriae are transient in nature and disappear in a week, causing no effect on visual outcomes. Persistent microstriae are a potential cause of suboptimal visual gain after keratorefractive surgery.

EPITHELIAL INGROWTH

Incidence

Epithelial ingrowth following SMILE has been observed in 0.5–0.66% cases.[1,2] The incidence is significantly less than LASIK, where epithelial ingrowth may be observed in 0.4–9.1% of cases (Figs. 9.2A and B).[9]

Pathophysiology

The presence of epithelial cells in the interface (beneath a LASIK flap or in the SMILE stromal pocket) is termed as epithelial ingrowth. Epithelial cells may enter the interface during excessive surgical manipulations or repeated interventions. These epithelial cells that enter the stromal interface die, most likely as a result of hypoxia, but continue to persist in the interface as the cornea does not contain phagocytic cells. This incites interface inflammation resulting in disruption of collagen fibrils and subsequent corneal haze. Epithelial

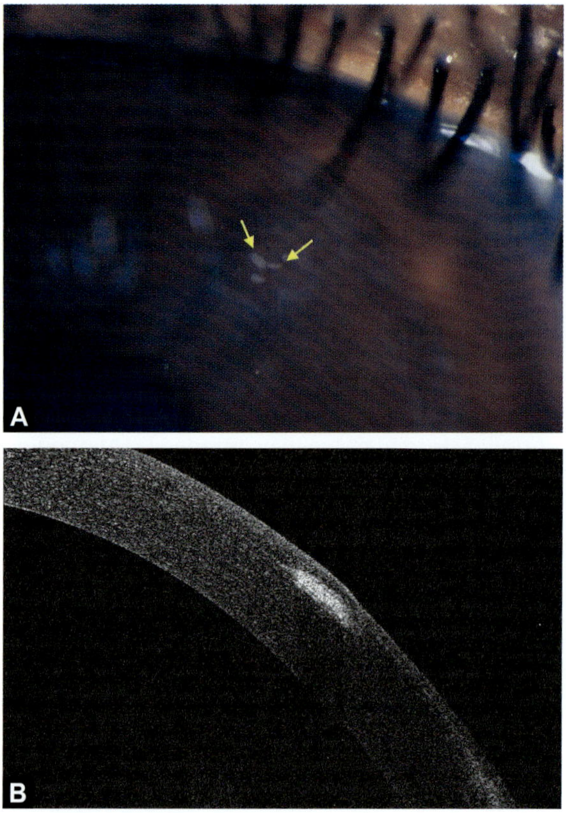

Figs. 9.2A and B: (A) Epithelial ingrowth with epithelial cell nests visible in the periphery (arrows: small epithelial nests). (B) Epithelial cell nests in the interface as observed on ASOCT.

ingrowth may be classified as "mild" (within 0.5–1.0 mm of the flap edge) or "clinically significant" (greater than 1 mm from the flap edge), depending on visual symptoms or discomfort.[10] However, the classification was developed for LASIK and no specific terminology exists for SMILE.

Predisposing Factors

The theoretical risk for the development of epithelial ingrowth is less in SMILE due to the smaller size of the incision. The following are the risk factors for development of epithelial ingrowth in a patient undergoing SMILE.

- *Epithelial defect during surgery*: Presence of epithelial defect especially near the incision site during the primary surgery increases the chances of postoperative epithelial ingrowth.
- *Anterior basement membrane dystrophy*: Patients with epithelial basement membrane disorders are at a higher risk of developing epithelial ingrowth.

- *Surgeon inexperience*: Surgery done by inexperienced surgeon resulting in excessive manipulations can cause corneal abrasions at the incision site, leading to an increased incidence of epithelial ingrowth.
- *Patient factors*: Various factors such as old age, diabetes mellitus, etc. may predispose to the formation of epithelial ingrowth.
- *Enhancement procedures*: Patients having undergone enhancement procedures with repeated handling of the interface and multiple flap-lifts are at a greater risk for developing epithelial ingrowth.

Management

The diagnosis of epithelial ingrowth is made clinically, and may be further confirmed on anterior segment optical coherence tomography (ASOCT) (Fig. 9.2B). The treatment of epithelial ingrowth depends on the clinical condition of the patient. Eyes with "mild" ingrowth are generally kept under observation. Clinically significant ingrowths causing visual symptoms, irregular astigmatism, and punctate staining warrant surgical intervention.

In a majority of cases of epithelial ingrowth after SMILE, small epithelial islands are noted at the incision site. These cases may be observed, since they may spontaneously resolve with time. More extensive localized epithelial ingrowth warranting intervention may be managed by scraping off the epithelial cells after opening the side cut. Frank epithelial ingrowth is rare due to the small incision size.

In cases of extensive epithelial ingrowth involving the visual axis, surgical treatment may be needed. The stromal cap may have to be converted into a flap in order to effectively scrape the epithelial cells from the interface. Flap edges may have to be sutured in recalcitrant cases or sealed with fibrin adhesives.[11]

Outcomes

Epithelial ingrowth in cases of SMILE may exist as epithelial cell-nests at the incision site which are non-progressive in a majority of cases, with no effect on visual outcomes.

UNDERCORRECTIONS, OVERCORRECTIONS, AND POSTOPERATIVE REGRESSION

Small incision lenticule extraction is a safe and effective procedure with good predictability in terms of refractive outcomes. The postoperative epithelial remodeling and stromal healing response is less in SMILE as compared to LASIK, therefore leading to more predictable outcomes.[12] The closed-chamber intrastromal surgical procedure in SMILE is independent of the environmental factors, further enhancing efficacy and predictability of the visual outcomes.

Incidence

The incidence of suboptimal visual gain mandating enhancement procedures is 2.1–4%.[13] This residual refractive error may result from undercorrection, overcorrection or regression, including residual and/or consecutive astigmatism.

Predisposing Factors

- *Age of the patient*: Age greater than 35 years is an important factor for postoperative regression. The biomechanical characteristics, stromal cellular response, and epithelial thickening response in older corneas is more unpredictable thus leading to a higher rate of regression.[14-16] The age-related increased stiffness of older corneas may affect the actual shape of the lenticule, thereby affecting refractive outcomes.[14]
- *Refractive error*: Eyes with preoperative manifest refraction spherical equivalent (MRSE) more than –6.00 D, preoperative myopia more than 6.00 D, and preoperative astigmatism more than 3.00 D are more likely to need enhancement surgery.[13] The chance of undercorrection is more in cases with higher astigmatism.[17]
- *Machine factors*: The standard company-advised nomogram has a tendency to undercorrect the refractive error.[18,19] Hjortdal et al. reported an undercorrection of 0.25 D in the standard SMILE nomogram, and steeper corneas were associated with undercorrection.

  In SMILE, the central lenticule thickness depends upon the amount of correction (1.00 D correction corresponds to approximately 13 microns tissue thickness).[20] Higher refractive corrections require a thicker lenticule to be extracted and result in abrupt changes in the corneal stromal surface.[21] Also, greater epithelial thickening is induced by increased magnitude of refractive errors. The greater stromal healing and corneal epithelial hyperplasia are mainly responsible for decreased predictability in patients with higher refractive errors.[21]

  Due to the absence of an eye tracker, the alignment in SMILE depends mainly on the patient's fixation and surgeon's application of a suction contact glass on the eye. This could be a potential cause of suboptimal astigmatic correction in some cases.
- *Suction loss*: Suction loss is an important risk factor for postoperative enhancement.[13] Retaining original centration may be very difficult during redocking, especially when the pupil is obscured by the intrastromal gas bubbles after the posterior lenticule surface is cut, resulting in an inaccurate anterior lenticule cut. Tissue edema may occur in areas where the laser had passed during repeated attempts of suction application and redocking, thereby affecting the accuracy of lenticule cut. Repeated laser cuts may distort the stromal collagen lamellae, leading to poorer refractive results.

- *Surgeon factors*: An inexperienced surgeon may experience an increased probability of suction loss and repeated docking attempts, thereby resulting in poor refractive outcomes.

Prevention

Careful patient selection for SMILE is of great importance. Those above 35 years of age should be dissuaded from surgery. It has been observed that an overcorrection is more common in low refractive errors and an undercorrection is more likely in high refractive errors. The surgeon may consider decreasing the attempted correction by 0.25 D for low myopia and increase the correction for high myopia. An optimization of the nomogram may help in minimizing postoperative undercorrections and overcorrections.[13]

Management

Various procedures have been described for enhancement in patients with suboptimal visual gain after SMILE. Refractive stability for a minimum period of at least 3 months should be ensured prior to any intervention.

Surface ablation in the form of PRK augmented with MMC is the simplest procedure to correct residual refractive error, although pain, slower recovery, and postoperative haze may limit the eventual outcomes.[22]

Secondary LASIK with a thinner flap, or secondary SMILE anterior or posterior to primary SMILE may also be considered.[23] A recent adaptation of SMILE software (Circle, Carl Zeiss Meditec AG) enables revision of the previously created cap by converting it into a larger diameter flap (with hinge), followed by excimer laser ablation.

Outcomes

The visual outcomes after enhancements are usually satisfactory. In a retrospective study done by Liu et al., 93% patients undergoing enhancement gained a vision of 6/12 to 6/6, with a mean residual spherical equivalent of 0.13 D.[13]

Postoperative haze may limit the visual outcomes after PRK, as observed in cases with irregular topography.[22]

IRREGULAR TOPOGRAPHY

Incidence

Irregular topography may be observed in 0.5–1% cases after SMILE.[1,2] It may result in poor visual gains, suboptimal quality of vision, ghost images, and monocular diplopia (Fig. 9.3).[2]

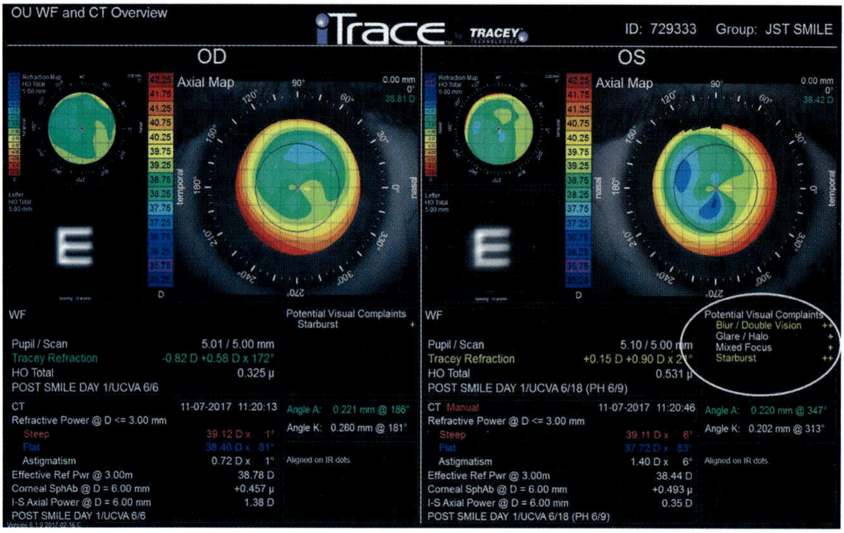

Fig. 9.3: Visual function analysis summary display showing potential visual complaints of blurred vision, glare, halos and starburst in the left eye after SMILE.

Predisposing Factors

The following factors may predispose to the development of irregular topography in a patient undergoing SMILE.

- *Increased intraoperative manipulations*: Difficulties in lenticule separation and extraction may predispose to the development of postoperative irregular corneal topography. Retained lenticule fragments also result in irregular astigmatism.[24]
- *Opaque bubble layer*: A dense opaque bubble layer is associated with increased adhesions and remnant tissue bridges; thereby leading to irregularities during the healing process.
- *Laser settings*: Laser settings with lower spot energy and closer spacing may result in irregular topography due to the irregular cleavage of tissue bridges. Optimization of laser settings is helpful in reducing this complication.
- *Surgeon factor*: Surgeon's inexperience leading to excess intraoperative manipulation may result in irregular interface and topographical abnormalities.

Management

In spite of the topographic irregularities, spontaneous improvement in vision is noted in majority of cases. Corneal or epithelial remodeling, stabilization of the tear film, and neuronal adaptation may be responsible for this improvement in vision.

In cases of non-improvement of vision, topography-guided PRK can be attempted. PRK may result in postoperative haze and prolonged postoperative recovery time. It should therefore be considered only after several months and in cases with significant visual symptoms.[1] Rigid gas permeable contact lens may be useful in some cases.

Outcomes

Topography-guided PRK resulted in improvement in visual acuity and remission of visual symptoms like halos and ghost images. Postoperative haze limits the visual outcomes, and concurrent MMC is advocated to achieve optimal results.[22]

OPTICAL ABERRATIONS

Incidence

Optical aberrations and dysphotic symptoms in the form of glare, halos, and ghost images may be observed after SMILE in 0.2–0.4% of cases (Figs. 9.4 to 9.6).[1,2]

Predisposing Factors

- *Surgeon factors*: Excessive intraoperative manipulations in the form of suction loss, multiple attempts of docking, and difficult lenticule dissection may lead to irregularity in the topography.
- *Retained lenticule*: Retained lenticule fragments may result in ghost images and monocular diplopia.
- *Decentered treatment*: Decentered treatment profile may induce higher-order aberrations (HOAs) like coma and trefoil which manifest as glare and halos.
- *Epithelial ingrowth*: Epithelial ingrowth in the stromal interface may cause irregular topography and hence cause visual symptoms.

Management

A comprehensive workup may help to identify the underlying cause for optical aberrations. ASOCT done in the postoperative period will help identify a retained stromal lenticule or epithelial ingrowth as a cause of monocular ghost images. Investigation to evaluate corneal topography, like Pentacam or Orbscan, should be done in all cases with visual symptoms to look for irregular topography. Abberometry should be done to look for the type of aberrations induced which would help in the management of the case (Figs. 9.4 to 9.6).

Mild cases may be observed, as enhancement procedures may not help in the resolution of HOAs. Topography-guided PRK seems to be a good option in patients with disabling symptoms due to irregular topography.[1]

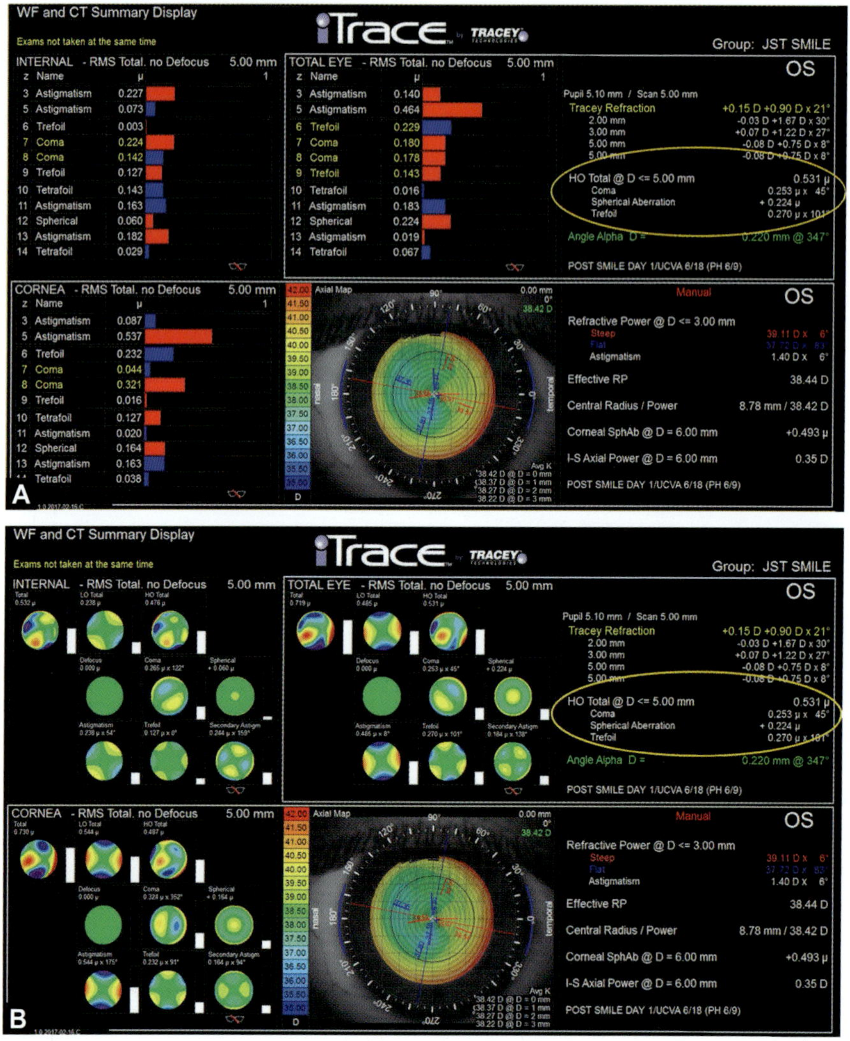

Figs. 9.4A and B: Higher order aberrations induced after SMILE. An increase in corneal aberrations, total aberrations and coma is observed on iTRACE system.

Outcomes

Remission of visual symptoms with good visual outcomes is observed in patients treated with topography-guided PRK. However, postoperative haze may limit the visual outcomes.[22]

DECENTERED TREATMENT

Accurate centration is of paramount importance in corneal refractive surgeries to achieve optimum visual outcomes. Decentered treatment may not

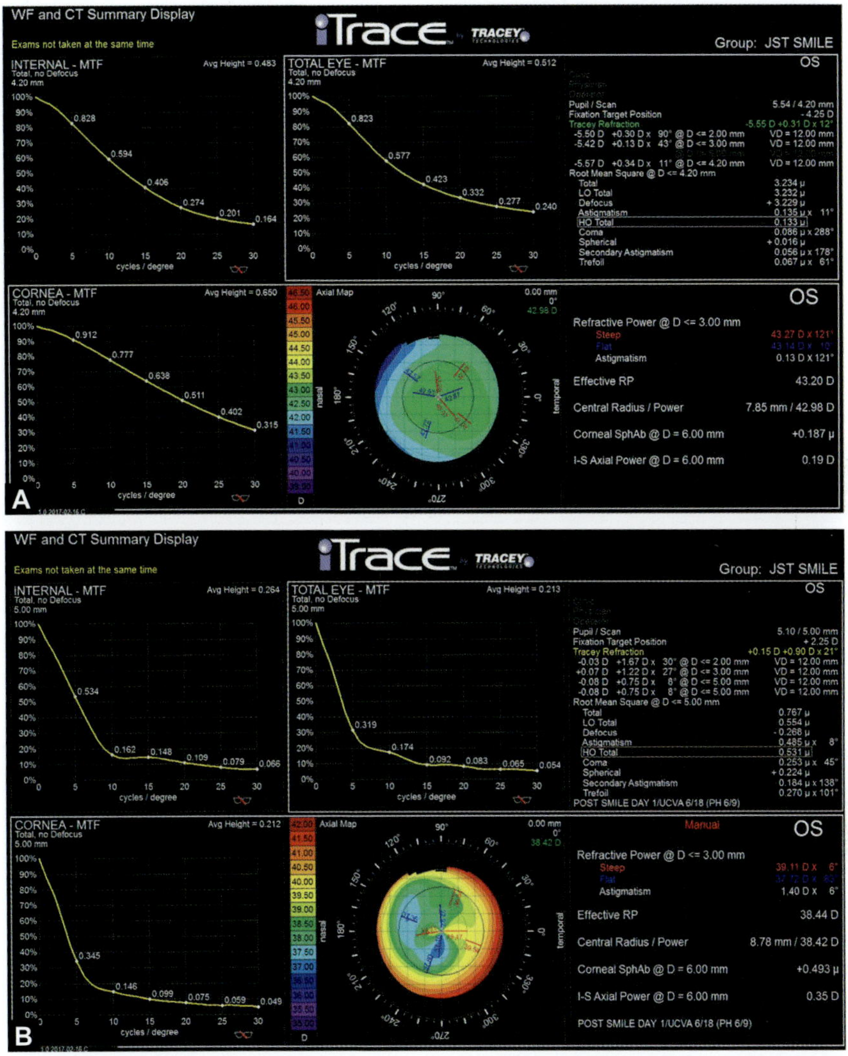

Figs. 9.5A and B: Worsening of modulation transfer function (MTF) observed after SMILE. (A) Preoperative MTF curves. (B) Postoperative MTF curves.

only cause suboptimal visual gain, but may also lead to many undesirable side effects, such as glare, halos, ghost images, and monocular diplopia (*see* Fig. 9.3).

Centration in corneal refractive surgeries may be with respect to the visual axis, the pupil center or the corneal vertex.[25] Anatomically, the corneal vertex is the point of maximum elevation when the patient is fixating on an internal target.[26] Corneal vertex centration has been observed to be superior to the entrance pupil centration, in terms of induced ocular aberrations and asphericity.[27,28]

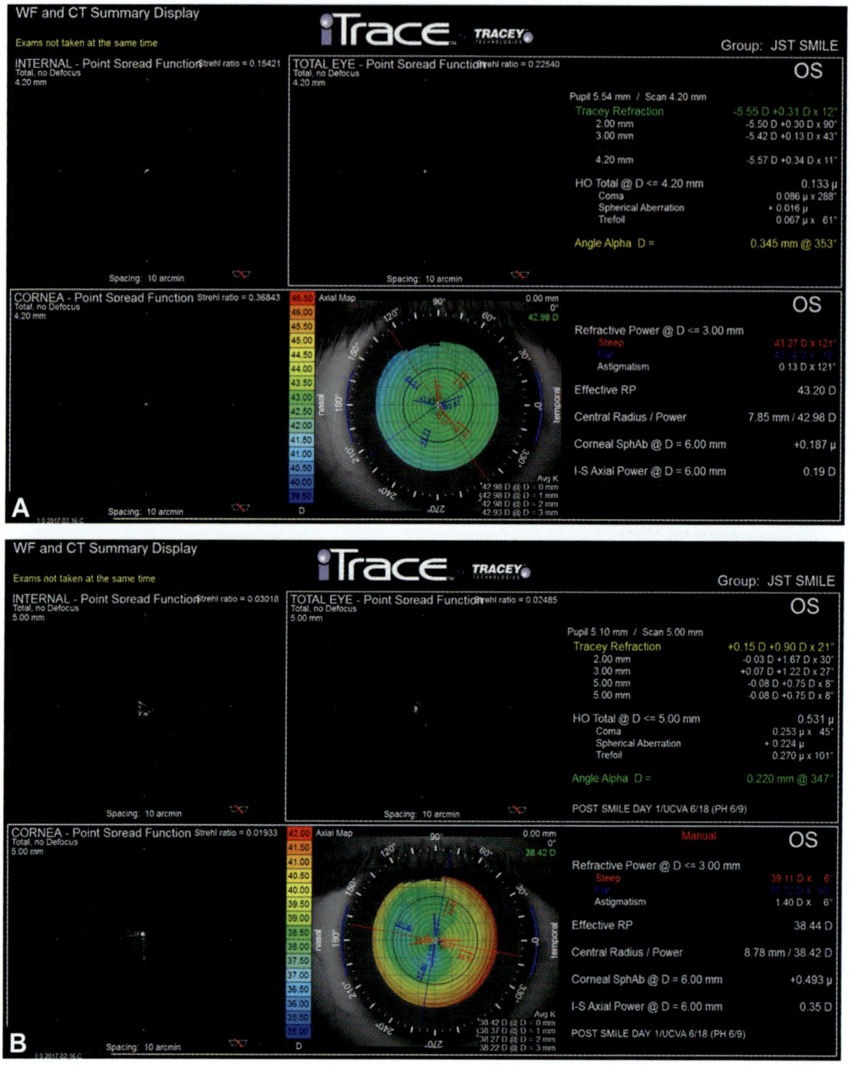

Figs. 9.6A and B: Worsening of point spread function (PSF) with increase in defocus observed after SMILE. (A) Preoperative PSF. (B) Postoperative PSF.

The postoperative topographic maps in SMILE exhibit a larger optical zone than topographic maps generated after femtosecond LASIK. Therefore, a decentered treatment in case of SMILE might cause only minimal impact on the patients' visual outcome.

Incidence

A decentration greater than 0.3 mm has been observed to induce HOAs with suboptimal visual quality.[29] In a study by Li et al., the ablation profile was decentered within 0.20 mm in 70% eyes, within 0.30 mm in 90% eyes, and within 0.50 mm in all eyes.[30]

Predisposing Factors

- *Patient factors*: Patients with a large angle kappa with a large disparity between the visual axis and corneal axis may be at a high risk of decentered treatment.
- *Surgeon factors*: The absence of an active eye tracker during the procedure makes it more surgeon-dependent, thereby increasing the risk of decentration in SMILE. Surgeon's inexperience during docking could be an important risk factor.

Prevention

Corneal vertex centration is deemed most accurate in corneal refractive surgeries. During the docking process, the patient is expected to focus at a blinking light. In patients with a small angle kappa, the visual axis and the corneal vertex tend to coincide, hence enabling a centered ablation; however, in patients with a large angle kappa, there might be an increased risk of decentered treatment. Thus patients with a large angle kappa may be excluded from the surgery.[30]

Absence of an active tracking system in SMILE makes the centration more surgeon-dependent. Decentration can occur during involuntary eye movements or when the surgeon attempts to correct an apparent decentration during the course of the treatment.

To ensure proper centration, the patient bed should be moved slowly. At the point when the cone touches the cornea, the corneal vertex should automatically fit the apex of the cone. Otherwise, a sudden generation of suction between the cornea and the suction cone may result in decentration.

In cases with eccentric docking, the suction should be released and the patient redocked in order to prevent an eccentric ablation.

Management

Care should be taken to avoid decentration during SMILE. Minimal decentration up to 0.3 mm from the corneal center does not cause visual symptoms and hence no intervention is needed. Surgical intervention should be considered in presence of dysphotic symptoms or loss of more than two lines of Snellen's visual acuity. Abberometry should be carried out in such patients to look for induced HOAs. Topography-guided PRK can be attempted in such cases; however, persistence of haze and prolonged postoperative recovery time may be seen with some patients.

Outcome

The decentration of the lenticule from the pupil center ranges from 0.07 mm to 0.3 mm after SMILE, as against 0.4 mm to 0.7 mm in LASIK.[29-32] It is observed that patients are more comfortable during SMILE and hence cooperate better.

The decentration has a greater influence on HOA in eyes with LASIK than SMILE, and the aberrations induced are majorly coma and trefoil. SMILE is better tolerated for horizontal displacement than LASIK but there exists a positive correlation between vertical displacement and HOA which could adversely affect visual outcomes.[32]

ECTASIA

Incidence

Corneal ectasia remains one of the most dreaded complications, which can occur months to years after uneventful keratorefractive surgery. Ectasia following SMILE is rare and there have been few case reports about the same.[33,34]

Pathophysiology

The biomechanical strength of the cornea is greater in its anterior layer due to stronger intralamellar collagen bonding. SMILE is essentially a flap-less surgery, where the lenticule is extracted through a small incision. This results in minimal disruption of peripheral collagen fibers compared to LASIK, thus providing superior corneal biomechanics.[35] However, the actual removal of corneal stromal tissue in SMILE does weaken the cornea to some extent, and hence there is always a theoretical risk of ectasia.

Predisposing Factors

The predisposing factors for ectasia in a case undergoing SMILE are similar to those in patients undergoing LASIK.

- *Keratoconus*: Patients with documented progressive ectatic disease like keratoconus are at a high risk of developing iatrogenic ectasia and hence should be dissuaded from surgery.
- *High myopia*: SMILE is currently limited to use in myopic patients up to 10.00 D. Correction of higher degree of refractive error will cause greater subtraction of tissue thereby causing greater weakening of the cornea.
- *Low residual stromal bed thickness*: A low residual stromal bed thickness (RSBT, <225–250 microns) is one of the most important factors predisposing to postsurgery ectasia. This could occur on account of preexisting thin cornea, excessive tissue removal on account of high myopia or thicker cap.

- *Preoperative topographic abnormalities*: Patients with suspicious preoperative corneal topography like forme fruste keratoconus or pellucid marginal degeneration are at a greater risk of postoperative ectasia.

Management

Though the risk of iatrogenic ectasia is less compared to LASIK, cautious selection of patients is of paramount importance. Thorough preoperative workup must be done in all cases to rule out preexisting manifest or forme-fruste ectasia. Collagen crosslinking (CXL) with SMILE is a promising option in patients with subclinical disease; however, long-term results are awaited.[36]

Outcomes

In a single case of unilateral corneal ectasia following SMILE, intrastromal corneal ring segment implantation with CXL was performed which helped to maintain the corrected distance visual acuity of 20/20.[34]

DIFFUSE LAMELLAR KERATITIS

Incidence

The incidence and clinical features of post-SMILE diffuse lamellar keratitis (DLK) have not been extensively evaluated. An incidence of 1.6% has been reported in a large retrospective case series, which is less than that reported after femtosecond LASIK.[37]

Pathophysiology

Diffuse lamellar keratitis is a sterile interface inflammatory response observed in the early postoperative period after refractive surgeries such as LASIK or SMILE. The onset is usually 1–2 days after surgery, though delayed onset has also been reported. The exact pathogenesis is unclear; however, various inciting factors have been implicated in the development of DLK, such as interface debris in the form of meibomian gland secretions, powder particles, blood, povidone-iodine, and bacterial endotoxins.[37,38]

Predisposing Factors

Various risk factors have been described in cases of post-SMILE DLK.

- *Lenticule thickness*: An increased incidence of DLK is observed with thinner lenticules.[37] The more intense inflammatory response may be attributed to the accumulation of intrastromal gas bubbles, which exert a compressive force and result in tightly pressed together anterior and posterior lenticule planes. Moreover, the surgical difficulty and excessive surgical manipulation required in thin lenticules may incite more inflammation.

- *Cap diameter*: A larger lenticule diameter is associated with the development of DLK.[37] This may be explained by the proximity of a larger lenticule to the limbal vasculature, which facilitates diffusion of inflammatory cells and mediators.
- *Interface debris*: Interface debris in the form of glove powder, mucous, wax, blood, povidone-iodine, epithelial cells, etc. incites inflammation and may result in DLK.
- *Surgeon factors*: Excessive surgical manipulation in technically challenging cases, or by an inexperienced surgeon incites interface inflammation and predisposes to the formation of DLK.
- *Laser settings*: High energy parameters predispose to interface inflammation and DLK.

Prevention

Smooth surgery with minimal intraoperative manipulations minimizes the incidence of DLK. Interface handling should be kept to a minimal. Thorough irrigation of the interface toward the end of surgery has been postulated to remove all debris. Laser energy settings should be optimal.

Management

The severity of DLK should be assessed, and may be graded according to the Linebarger classification described for post-LASIK DLK.[39] Mild cases are treated with frequent instillation of topical corticosteroids. Severe cases require both oral and topical corticosteroids along with interface irrigation, and the cap may need to be converted into a flap.[40]

Outcomes

Diffuse lamellar keratitis observed after SMILE is usually mild in severity, and good visual and anatomical outcomes are observed. Majority of the cases resolve within 1–2 weeks of institution of treatment.

INFECTIOUS KERATITIS

Incidence

The incidence of infectious keratitis ranges from 0.02% to 0.2% after surface ablation procedures and approximately 0.03% after LASIK.[41-43] The incidence among SMILE patients is approximately 0.3%.[1,44] There has only been a single case report of bilateral infectious keratitis following SMILE.[45]

Predisposing Factors and Causative Agents

A variety of organisms have been identified in infectious keratitis following LASIK procedures. Early-onset infections (occurring within 2 weeks of surgery) are mainly caused by gram-positive bacteria, particularly staphylococcal and streptococcal species, whereas atypical mycobacteria and fungi are implicated in late-onset infections, occurring from 2 weeks to 3 months postsurgery.[46]

The potential sources of infections in these cases could be surgeons' hands, contaminated surgical instruments, environmental factors, and periocular flora.

Presenting Features

The patient may present with a plethora of symptoms ranging from ocular irritation to intense pain, photophobia, tearing and purulent discharge, and diminution of vision. Slit-lamp examination will reveal infiltrates in the interface, with or without associated epithelial defect.

Management

Thorough microbiological workup prior to starting of therapy is of paramount importance in such cases. As the infection is generally restricted to the stromal pocket, obtaining microbiological sample by conventional scraping method is difficult. In such cases, the stromal pocket should be opened and sample for microbiological analysis should be taken directly from the infective lesion. Irrigation of the stromal pocket with fortified antibiotics may allow better delivery of drug and hence hasten the recovery. Empirical topical antibiotics should be promptly administered, and can later be amended according to culture sensitivity reports. Topical steroids can be started early in the course in cases of proven bacterial keratitis as it would help to reduce the inflammation and hence reduce scarring. Serial ASOCT imaging can be done to look for infiltrates in the interface, as well as document the progress. Stromal cap amputation or therapeutic penetrating keratoplasty may be needed in fulminant cases.

Outcome

Majority of cases presented with interface infiltrates where specific organisms could not be isolated, but patients responded to empirical antibacterial therapy.

CONCLUSION

In conclusion, although SMILE is a promising technique for the correction of myopia and myopic astigmatism with predictable and efficient refractive and visual outcomes, complications can occur. Most of them are observed in the learning curve of the technique with favorable resolution, and majority are mild and do not affect final visual outcome.

REFERENCES

1. Ivarsen A, Asp S, Hjortdal J. Safety and complications of more than 1500 small-incision lenticule extraction procedures. Ophthalmology. 2014;121(4):822-8.
2. Moshirfar M, McCaughey MV, Reinstein DZ, et al. Small-incision lenticule extraction. J Cataract Refract Surg. 2015;41(3):652-65.
3. Dong Z, Zhou X, Wu J, et al. Small incision lenticule extraction (SMILE) and femtosecond laser LASIK: comparison of corneal wound healing and inflammation. Br J Ophthalmol. 2014;98(2):263-9.
4. Riau AK, Angunawela RI, Chaurasia SS, et al. Early corneal wound healing and inflammatory responses after refractive lenticule extraction (ReLEx). Invest Ophthalmol Vis Sci. 2011;52(9):6213-21.
5. Agca A, Ozgurhan EB, Yildirim Y, et al. Corneal backscatter analysis by in vivo confocal microscopy: fellow eye comparison of small incision lenticule extraction and femtosecond laser-assisted LASIK. J Ophthalmol. 2014;2014:265012.
6. Vestergaard AH, Grønbech KT, Grauslund J, et al. Subbasal nerve morphology, corneal sensation and tear film evaluation after refractive femtosecond laser lenticule extraction. Graefes Arch Clin Exp Ophthalmol. 2013;251(11):2591-600.
7. Mohamed-Noriega K, Riau AK, Lwin NC, et al. Early corneal nerve damage and recovery following small incision lenticule extraction (SMILE) and laser in situ keratomileusis (LASIK). Invest Ophthalmol Vis Sci. 2014;55(3):1823-34.
8. Kamiya K, Igarashi A, Ishii R, et al. Early clinical outcomes, including efficacy and endothelial cell loss, of refractive lenticule extraction using a 500 kHz femtosecond laser to correct myopia. J Cataract Refract Surg. 2012;38(11):1996-2002.
9. Kamburoglu G, Ertan A. Epithelial ingrowth after femtosecond laser-assisted in situ keratomileusis. Cornea. 2008;27(10):1122-5.
10. Rapuano CJ. Management of epithelial ingrowth after laser in situ keratomileusis on a tertiary care cornea service. Cornea. 2010;29(3):307-13.
11. Thulasi P, Kim SW, Shetty R, et al. Recalcitrant epithelial ingrowth after SMILE treated with a hydrogel ocular sealant. J Refract Surg. 2015;31(12):847-50.
12. Luft N, Ring MH, Dirisamer M, et al. Corneal epithelial remodeling induced by small incision lenticule extraction (SMILE). Invest Ophthalmol Vis Sci. 2016;57(9):176-83.
13. Liu YC, Rosman M, Mehta JS. Enhancement after small-incision lenticule Extraction Incidence, risk factors, and outcomes. Ophthalmology. 2017;124(6): 813-21.
14. Hjortdal JØ, Vestergaard AH, Ivarsen A, et al. Predictors for the outcome of small incision lenticule extraction for myopia. J Refract Surg. 2012;28(12):865-71.
15. Netto MV, Mohan RR, Ambrósio R Jr, et al. Wound healing in the cornea: a review of refractive surgery complications and new prospects for therapy. Cornea. 2005;24(5):509-22.
16. Reinstein DZ, Archer TJ, Gobbe M. Improved effectiveness of transepithelial PTK versus topography-guided ablation for stromal irregularities masked by epithelial compensation. J Refract Surg. 2013;29(8):526-33.
17. Ivarsen A, Hjortdal J. Correction of myopic astigmatism with small lenticule extraction. J Refract Surg. 2014;30(4):240-7.
18. Ganesh S. Refining results with SMILE: tips and tricks. In: Sekundo W (Ed). Small Incision Lenticule Extraction (SMILE): Basic Principles, Current Techniques, Complication Management and Future Concepts. New York: Springer; 2015. pp. 68-73.

19. Ibrahim O, Abdalla M, Saeed A, et al. SMILE for correction of very high myopic (higher than e10D). In: Sekundo W (Ed). Small Incision Lenticule Extraction (SMILE): Basic Principles, Current Techniques, Complication Management and Future Concepts. New York: Springer; 2015. pp. 185-91.
20. Bischoff M, Strobrawa G. Femtosecond laser keratomes for small incision lenticule extraction. In: Sekundo W (Ed). Small Incision Lenticule Extraction (SMILE): Basic Principles, Current Techniques, Complication Management and Future Concepts. New York: Springer; 2015. pp. 6-11.
21. Hersh PS, Schein OD, Steinert R. Characteristics influencing outcomes of excimer laser photorefractive keratectomy. Summit Photorefractive Keratectomy Phase III Study Group. Ophthalmology. 1996;103(11):1962-9.
22. Ivarsen A, Hjortdal JØ. Topography-guided photorefractive keratectomy for irregular astigmatism after small incision lenticule extraction. J Refract Surg. 2014;30(6):429-32.
23. Reinstein DZ, Carp GI, Archer TJ, et al. Outcomes of small incision lenticule extraction (SMILE) in low myopia. J Refract Surg. 2014;30(12):812-8.
24. Dong Z, Zhou X. Irregular astigmatism after femtosecond laser refractive lenticule extraction. J Cataract Refract Surg. 2013;39(6):952-4.
25. Wu L, Zhou X, Chu R, et al. Photoablation centration on the corneal optical center in myopic LASIK using AOV excimer laser. Eur J Ophthalmol. 2009;19(6):923-9.
26. Park CY, Oh SY, Chuck RS. Measurement of angle kappa and centration in refractive surgery. Curr Opin Ophthalmol. 2012;23(4):269-75.
27. Reinstein DZ, Archer TJ, Gobbe M. Is topography-guided ablation profile centered on the corneal vertex better than wavefront-guided ablation profile centered on the entrance pupil? J Refract Surg. 2012;28(2):139-43.
28. Arbelaez MC, Vidal C, Arba-Mosquera S. Clinical outcomes of corneal vertex versus central pupil references with aberration free ablation strategies and LASIK. Invest Ophthalmol Vis Sci. 2008;49(12):5287-94.
29. Lee SB, Hwang BS, Lee J. Effects of decentration of photorefractive keratectomy on the induction of higher order wavefront aberrations. J Refract Surg. 2010; 26(10):731-43.
30. Li M, Zhao J, Miao H, et al. Mild decentration measured by a Scheimpflug camera and its impact on visual quality following SMILE in the early learning curve. Invest Ophthalmol Vis Sci. 2014;55(6):3886-92.
31. Liu M, Sun Y, Wang D, et al. Decentration of optical zone center and its impact on visual outcomes following smile. Cornea. 2015;34(4):392-7.
32. Yu Y, Zhang W, Cheng X, et al. Impact of treatment decentration on higher-order aberrations after SMILE. J Ophthalmol. 2017;2017:9575723.
33. El-Naggar MT. Bilateral ectasia after femtosecond laser assisted small-incision lenticule extraction. J Cataract Refract Surg. 2015;41(4):884-8.
34. Sachdev G, Sachdev MS, Sachdev R, et al. Unilateral corneal ectasia following small-incision lenticule extraction. J Cataract Refract Surg. 2015;41(9):2014-8.
35. Sinha Roy A, Duppus WJ Jr, Roberts CJ. Comparison of biomechanical effects of small-incision lenticule extraction and laser in situ keratomileusis: finite element analysis. J Cataract Refract Surg. 2014;40(6):971-80.
36. Ganesh S, Brar S. Clinical outcomes of small incision lenticule extraction with accelerated cross-linking (ReLEx SMILE Xtra) in patients with thin corneas and borderline topography. J Ophthalmol. 2015;2015:263412.
37. Zhao J, He L, Yao P, et al. Diffuse lamellar keratitis after small-incision lenticule extraction. J Cataract Refract Surg. 2015;41(2):400-7.

38. Hoffman RS, Fine IH, Packer M. Incidence and outcomes of LASIK with diffuse lamellar keratitis treated with topical and oral corticosteroids. J Cataract Refract Surg. 2003;29(3):451-6.
39. Linebarger EJ, Hardten DR, Lindstrom RL. Diffuse lamellar keratitis: diagnosis and management. J Cataract Refract Surg. 2000;26(7):1072-7.
40. Steinert RF, Swami AU. Diffuse interface keratitis. Rev Ophthalmol. 2001;8:46-52.
41. De Rojas V, Llovet F, Martınez M, et al. Infectious keratitis in 18,651 laser surface ablation procedures. J Cataract Refract Surg. 2011;37(10):1822-31.
42. Wroblewski KJ, Pasternak JF, Bower KS, et al. Infectious keratitis after photorefractive keratectomy in the United States Army and Navy. Ophthalmology. 2006;113(4):520-5.
43. Llovet F, de Rojas V, Interlandi E, et al. Infectious keratitis in 204,586 LASIK procedures. Ophthalmology. 2010;117(2):232-8.
44. Vestergaard A, Ivarsen A, Asp S, et al. Small-incision lenticule extraction for moderate to high myopia: predictability, safety and patient satisfaction. J Cataract Refract Surg. 2012;38(11):2003-10.
45. Chehaibou I, Sandali O, Ameline B, et al. Bilateral infectious keratitis after small incision lenticule extraction. J Cataract Refract Surg. 2016;42(4):626-30.
46. Chang MA, Jain S, Azar DT. Infections following laser in situ keratomileusis: an integration of the published literature. Surv Ophthalmol. 2004;49(3):269-80.

Chapter 10

Post-SMILE Enhancement and Retreatment

Manpreet Kaur, Jeewan S Titiyal

INTRODUCTION

The safety and efficacy of small incision lenticule extraction (SMILE) is well established with 77% of eyes achieving refractive correction within ±0.5 D of the intended target, and 95% of eyes within ±1 D of the intended target.[1] Post-SMILE enhancement may still be needed in 2.7–4% of cases with suboptimal visual gain, residual refractive errors and postoperative regression.[2,3] Moreover, cases with abandoned surgical procedure and retained lenticules also require retreatment. A major drawback of SMILE is the difficulty associated with repeating the surgical procedure in cases requiring retreatment.

A repeat SMILE is not advisable owing to the technical difficulties associated with identifying the original lenticule plane and creating a second lenticule. Creation of a second lenticule may interfere with the incisions of the initial SMILE procedure, thereby creating loose stromal fragments and subsequent difficulties in lenticule dissection as well as extraction. Though it may be possible to perform a second procedure either more superficially in the cap or deeper to the original plane, further clinical testing and validation of the technique will be required.

The various surgical modalities available for post-SMILE enhancement or retreatment include surface ablation, thin-flap laser-assisted in situ keratomileusis (LASIK) and the circle pattern of VisuMax laser.[2-6] A sub-cap lenticule extraction has been tried, however, its efficacy and surgical protocol is not yet established.[7] In this chapter, we will review the indications for retreatment, risk factors, various available and upcoming surgical modalities and their outcomes.

INDICATIONS

A postsurgical enhancement may be required in cases with primary undercorrection, primary overcorrection or postsurgical refractive regression. Moreover, enhancement may also be needed in cases with irregular astigmatism as a result of decentered ablation, difficult lenticule dissection or partially retained lenticule fragments.

Retreatment is needed in cases with abandoned primary surgical procedure. A partially created lenticule may be present in cases with intraoperative suction loss. A completely retained lenticule may be present in cases with difficult lenticule dissection and failure to extract the lenticule.

INCIDENCE

The incidence of post-SMILE enhancement is 2.7–4%.[2,3] We have observed a retreatment incidence of 3% as a result of intraoperative suction loss and completely retained lenticule.[8]

RISK FACTORS

Various risk factors have been identified that increase the incidence of retreatment and enhancements.[3,8]

Patient Age

Age of more than 35 years at the time of primary surgery is associated with a higher incidence of post-SMILE retreatment.[3] This may be attributed to the different wound healing response after refractive surgery in older individuals. The unpredictable stromal cellular response and a stronger epithelial thickening response observed with increasing age is responsible for postoperative regression.[9,10]

Laterality

An increased incidence of post-SMILE enhancement has been observed in right eyes.[3] The right eye was the dominant eye in these cases, and operated before the left eye in bilateral surgeries. Patients may be more sensitive to minor refractive errors in their dominant eye, thereby explaining the higher incidence of enhancement.

Magnitude of Refractive Error

Manifest refraction spherical equivalent (MRSE) of more than 6.0 D is associated with a greater risk of retreatment. Increased wound remodeling and epithelial thickening is observed in higher refractive errors, resulting in postoperative regression.[11]

Suction Loss

Intraoperative suction loss is a significant risk factor for post-SMILE enhancement and retreatment.[3] Redocking and completing SMILE after suction loss may result in creation of collagen lamellae distortion and irregular dissection planes. Centration may not be accurate during redocking, resulting in eccentric lenticules. Moreover, difficulties may be experienced during lenticule dissection resulting in suboptimal visual outcomes.[1] Abandoned surgical procedures after suction loss and partially created lenticules also require retreatment.[8]

Surgeon Factors

Surgeon's inexperience may result in a myriad of complications during the learning curve, which may lead to irregular astigmatism, suboptimal visual outcomes and need for retreatment.[1,8]

Difficult Lenticule Dissection

Excessive surgical manipulation in cases with difficult lenticule extraction may result in persistent interface haze and posterior stromal damage.[8] Various factors predispose to difficult lenticule dissection, as detailed in Chapter 8 "Intraoperative Complications in Small Incision Lenticule Extraction". It may result in postoperative irregular astigmatism or retention of lenticules, for which retreatment is required.

SURGICAL MODALITIES

A thorough refractive workup is essential before proceeding for retreatment. Comprehensive details of the previous surgery may help guide the choice of the second refractive procedure. Each surgery has its own pros and cons, which should be weighed on a case-to-case basis to determine the decision regarding the optimal technique.

Preoperative Considerations

A thorough refractive workup should be undertaken before planning a retreatment. The details of the previous surgery, magnitude of refractive correction, residual stromal bed thickness (RSBT) and any intraoperative or postoperative complications should be noted. A cycloplegic and manifest refraction should be undertaken.

An anterior segment optical coherence tomography (ASOCT) may be undertaken to determine the cap thickness as well as the RSBT.

It is advisable to allow a time period of at least 3 months to elapse before undertaking retreatment in order to ensure refractive stability.

Decision-making

The options for retreatment include surface ablation, flap-based excimer laser ablation or circle pattern of VisuMax laser. A sub-cap lenticule extraction has been tried, though further clinical testing is required before its widespread usage. The various factors guiding decision-making are described below and in Flowchart 10.1.

Flowchart 10.1: Decision-making in post-SMILE retreatment.

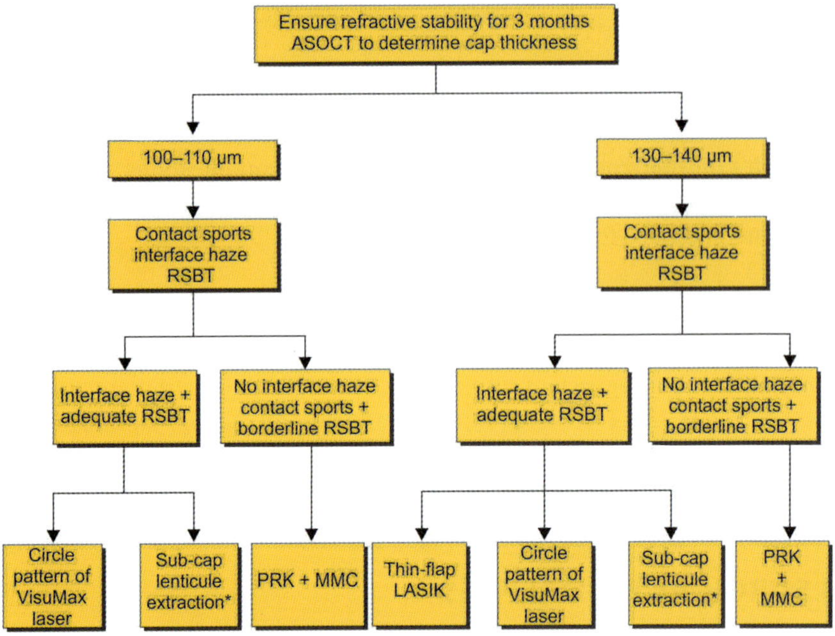

* Further clinical testing required for this technique.
(ASOCT: Anterior segment optical coherence tomography; RSBT: Residual stromal bed thickness; PRK: Photorefractive keratectomy; MMC: Mitomycin C).

- *Cap thickness*: The cap thickness during the primary SMILE procedure should be ascertained. In cases with a thick cap (130–140 µm), a thin-flap LASIK can be undertaken as a secondary procedure. In cases with a thin cap (100–110 µm), a LASIK flap may intersect with the previous interface, and photorefractive keratectomy (PRK) may be a better option.
- *Interface haze*: PRK is associated with postoperative haze. In cases with residual interface haze after the primary surgery, PRK may be avoided as it can further worsen the haze and result in suboptimal visual outcomes.
- *Residual stromal bed thickness*: In cases with a borderline RSBT after the initial SMILE surgery, further ablation beneath the SMILE interface should be avoided. In-the-cap ablation such as a thin-flap LASIK or PRK are preferred over a sub-cap lenticule extraction or a circle pattern of VisuMax laser.
- *Patient factors*: Patients involved in contact sports will not prefer a flap-based procedure, and PRK may be a better choice in such cases.
- *Surgeon factors*: The expertise of the operating surgeon in various techniques may determine the choice of secondary procedure.

Surgical Technique

The different surgical options available for retreatment are described below and summarized in Table 10.1.

Table 10.1: Surgical modalities for retreatment after small incision lenticule extraction (SMILE)

Surgical procedure	*Technique*	*Advantages*	*Disadvantages*	*Clinical outcomes*
Photorefractive keratectomy (PRK)	Transepithelial/epithelium off Mitomycin C (0.02%) for 60 seconds after excimer laser ablation	Flapless	Postoperative haze	Satisfactory outcomes in majority Postoperative haze in irregular astigmatism
Thin-flap LASIK	Flap diameter 7.9–8.1 mm (larger than cap diameter) Nasal hinge (width ~3.5 mm) Flap thickness 90–100 µm	No postoperative haze Above the SMILE interface- avoids multiple dissection planes	Flap-related complications	Satisfactory outcomes
Circle pattern (cap to flap)	Pattern D (lamellar ring adjacent to the SMILE pocket cut, at the same depth of the pocket)	Utilizes original SMILE interface—Minimizes risk of multiple dissection planes Can extract retained lenticule No postoperative haze	Flap-related complications	Satisfactory outcomes
Sub-cap lenticule extraction	Modified repeat SMILE-Original SMILE pocket cut acts as superior border of new lenticule	Flapless	Technically challenging Thin lenticules may be difficult to extract—risk of cap tears	Satisfactory outcomes Requires further clinical testing

(LASIK: Laser-assisted in situ keratomileusis).

Photorefractive Keratectomy

Photorefractive keratectomy is excimer-laser surface ablation and has the advantage of not interfering with the previous SMILE interface during retreatment. The corneal epithelium may be removed with the application of 20% absolute alcohol for 45 seconds.[3] Alternatively, a transepithelial PRK may be performed.[12] An excimer laser ablation is performed with an optical zone of 6.5 mm. Postoperative haze may be a problem, hence, topical mitomycin C (MMC) application is recommended after excimer laser ablation. MMC (0.02%) application for 60 seconds is effective in preventing postoperative haze after post-SMILE enhancement with PRK.[3] Topography-guided PRK may be performed in cases with irregular astigmatism.

Visual outcomes are usually satisfactory; however, suboptimal outcomes with postoperative haze have been experienced in the treatment of irregular astigmatism with topography-guided PRK.[12]

Photorefractive keratectomy has the advantage of retaining the flapless nature of surgery. Moreover, it does not interfere with the previous SMILE interface and can be safely undertaken in all cases irrespective of cap thickness.

Thin-flap LASIK

In cases with a thick cap of 130–140 µm, a thin-flap LASIK can be performed within the initial cap (Figs. 10.1A and B and 18). In cases with a thin cap of 100–110 µm, the LASIK flap may intersect with the previous cap cut. This will lead to the creation of multiple dissection planes and increase the risk of

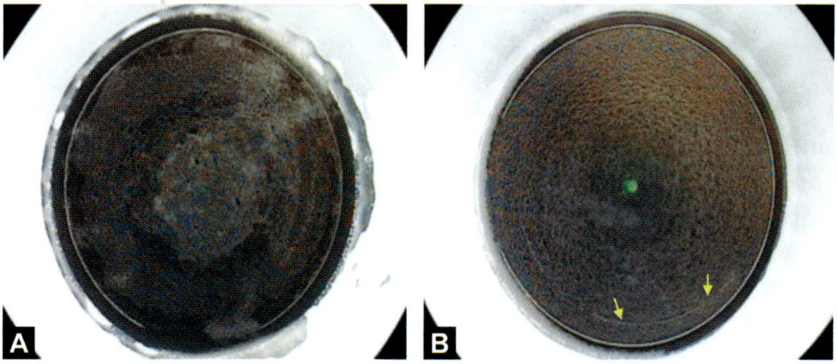

Figs. 10.1A and B: Thin-flap LASIK as retreatment after small incision lenticule extraction (SMILE). (A) Superior hinge-based flap in a case of intraoperative suction loss. Superior hinge was selected since suction loss occurred before creation of side cut; (B) Nasal hinge-based flap in a case of post-SMILE retreatment. Previous superior side cut is visible with localized scarring (arrows: previous cap side cut).
(LASIK: Laser-assisted in situ keratomileusis).

an irregular interface, loose stromal fragments as well as cause difficulties in lifting the flap. LASIK should be avoided in cases with a thin cap to prevent suboptimal visual outcomes.

The flap settings should be customized in post-SMILE cases to avoid the initial incisions. The flap diameter should be larger than the SMILE cap diameter and a nasal position of the hinge should be planned away from the site of the initial side cut.[8] The flap thickness should be set at 90–100 microns. We performed thin-flap LASIK in three cases (suction loss in one case and retained lenticules in two cases) and preferred a 7.9–8.1 mm diameter flap with a hinge diameter of 3.45–3.53 mm and flap thickness of 90 microns. The hinge position was superior in a case with suction loss, since a cap side cut was not present. In cases with retained lenticule, a nasal hinge was planned away from the initial side cut. Optimal visual outcomes could be achieved in all cases, with postoperative uncorrected distance visual acuity of 20/20.

In cases with a thin-cap, a femtosecond laser can potentially be used to create a side cut only, to convert the cap into a flap; however, this will limit the optical zone for excimer laser ablation. A deep LASIK flap extending beyond the initial cap is also a potential option in thin caps; however, it may still interfere with previous incisions and the RSBT may not be adequate for a thick flap.

On the flip side, performing a thin-flap LASIK negates the biomechanical stability of the primary procedure, and all the flap-related complications may possibly be encountered.

Circle Pattern of VisuMax Laser

A circle pattern of VisuMax laser (Carl Zeiss Meditec AG) has been developed to convert the original SMILE cap into a complete flap (19).[4,6] The procedure consists of creating a lamellar ring, a side cut and a junction cut (Figs. 10.2A and B). The lamellar ring is an incision plane encircling the original cap cut. A side cut with a hinge is created around the new incision plane, and the junction cut joins the original cap with the new incision plane to create one larger surface.

The flap thus created can be easily lifted and enhancement can be done using excimer laser ablation. Alternatively, a completely retained lenticule can be removed after lifting the flap.

Four patterns of circle cut have been described, based upon the plane of the lamellar ring and the position of side cut and junction cut (Figs. 10.3A to D).[4,6] Pattern A involves the creation of a side cut within the SMILE pocket cut, without an intervening lamellar ring or junction cut. The side cut borders on the outer diameter of the lamellar cut that extends to the surface of the cornea and the angle of the side cut impacts the diameter of the side cut on the surface. Pattern B creates a lamellar ring, posterior to the

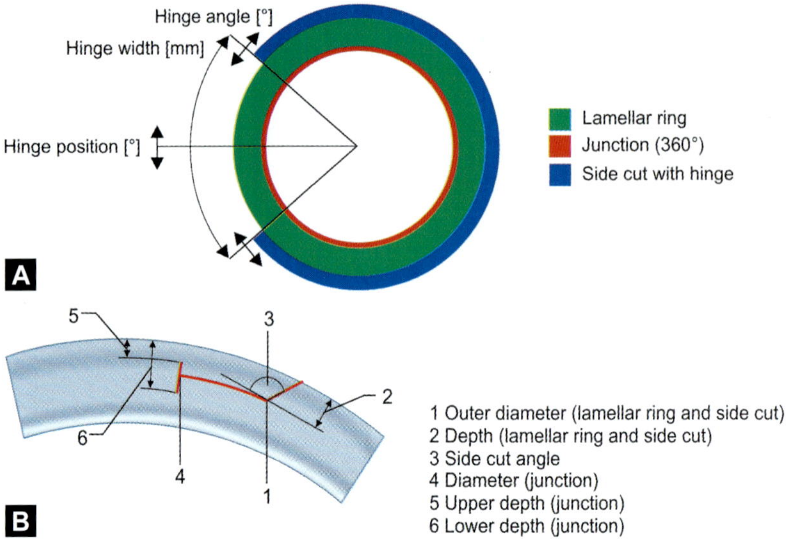

Figs. 10.2A and B: Circle pattern of VisuMax laser to convert the cap into a flap with junction, lamellar and side cut.

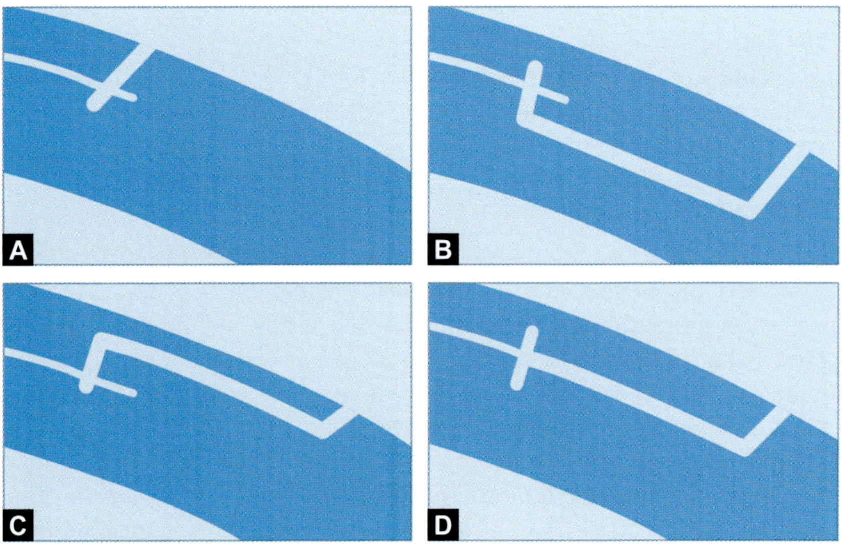

Figs. 10.3A to D: Four variants of circle pattern of VisuMax laser. (A) Pattern A (side cut only): Only the side cut of the flap is generated; (B) Pattern B: Lamellar ring deeper than existing incision and junction cut to upper side; (C) Pattern C: Lamellar ring higher than existing incision and junction cut to lower side; (D) Pattern D: Lamellar ring with same depth as existing incision and junction cut in each direction.

SMILE pocket cut. Pattern C creates a lamellar ring, anterior to the SMILE pocket cut. Pattern D creates a lamellar ring adjacent to the SMILE pocket

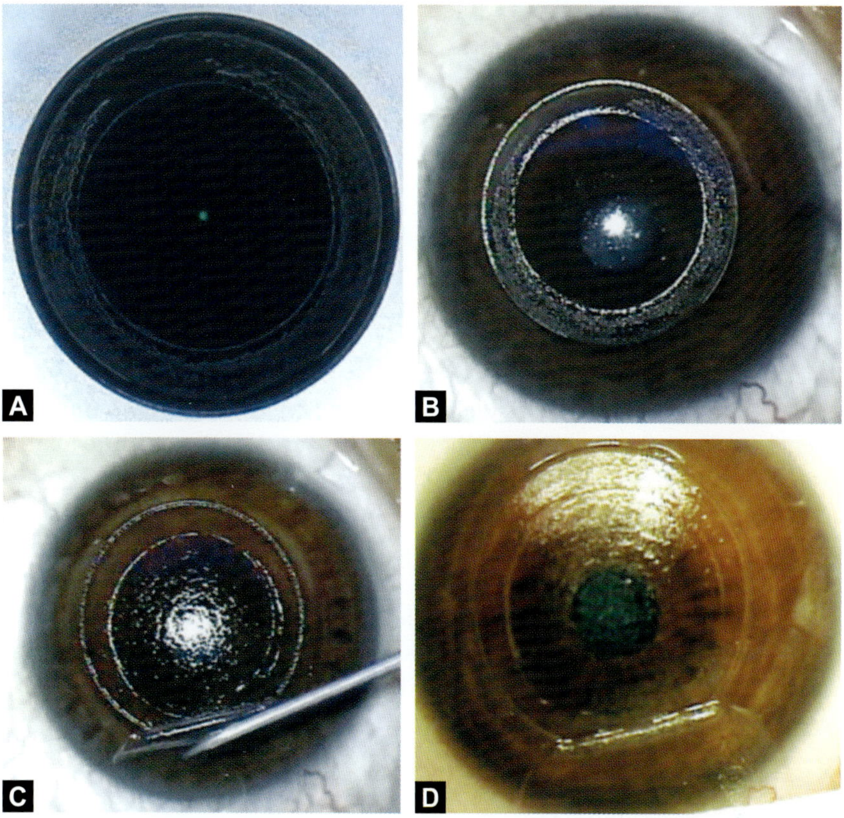

Figs. 10.4A to D: Post-SMILE enhancement using circle pattern of VisuMax laser. (A and B) Femtosecond laser delivery to create circle pattern "D" of VisuMax laser; (C) Flap created by the circle pattern is lifted with Seibel spatula; (D) Excimer laser ablation performed after lifting the flap.

cut, at the same depth of the pocket. Pattern D has been observed to be the most optimal pattern with the easiest flap lifting in cases of post-SMILE retreatment (Figs. 10.4A to D).[4]

The advantage of circle pattern is the elimination of the risk of multiple dissection planes in the optical zone, since the previous interface is extended to lift the flap. Moreover, in cases with a completely retained lenticule, the lenticule can be peeled off after lifting the flap. However, flap-related complications may occur.

Sub-cap Lenticule Extraction

Sub-cap lenticule extraction is a modified repeat SMILE procedure, which is performed at the same depth as the first procedure without the upper cut.[7] The previous interface acts as the superior border of the new lenticule. The advantages of a flap-less procedure are preserved; however, the surgery may be technically challenging in cases with a thin lenticule. The technique has been used to successfully perform a post-SMILE enhancement of –1.0 DS –1.0 DC@ 5° in a 53-year-old female.[7] Further clinical trials are required to establish the safety and efficacy of this procedure.

CLINICAL OUTCOMES

Satisfactory visual outcomes can be achieved in a majority of cases that undergo retreatment with any of the available surgical options.[1-3,6,8] Successful enhancement has also been reported after re-lifting the flap in a case of femtosecond lenticule extraction (FLEx) and performing excimer laser ablation.[13] Postoperative haze may limit the visual recovery in cases undergoing PRK. Optimal results may also not be achieved after enhancement in cases with irregular astigmatism. A repeat SMILE procedure may be promising; however, further clinical trials are required to establish its safety and efficacy.

Biomechanical weakening has been reported after retreatment in an experimental study, with a decrease in the elastic module of the eye.[5] LASIK had the most pronounced negative effect on corneal biomechanical integrity followed by repeat SMILE and PRK. Collagen cross-linking significantly increased the elastic modulus of the cornea and may be beneficial when used in conjunction with different refractive procedures for enhancement.[5]

CONCLUSION

Retreatment after SMILE may be required in cases with undercorrection, overcorrection, regression, suction loss or retained lenticules. Various surgical options are available such as PRK, thin-flap LASIK and circle pattern to convert the cap to flap. Satisfactory visual outcomes can be achieved in a majority of cases, though the advantages of a flapless procedure may not be retained. A repeat SMILE procedure is technically challenging owing to the risk of multiple dissection planes. However, a sub-cap lenticule extraction has been successfully tried and in the future, it may be possible to perform a repeat SMILE procedure for enhancement.

REFERENCES

1. Ivarsen A, Asp S, Hjortdal J. Safety and complications of more than 1500 small-incision lenticule extraction procedures. Ophthalmology. 2014;121:822-8.
2. Reinstein DZ, Carp GI, Archer TJ, et al. Outcomes of small incision lenticule extraction (SMILE) in low myopia. J Refract Surg. 2014;30:812-8.
3. Liu YC, Rosman M, Mehta JS. Enhancement after small-incision lenticule extraction: incidence, risk factors, and outcomes. Ophthalmology. 2017;124:813-21.
4. Riau AK, Ang HP, Lwin NC, et al. Comparison of four different VisuMax circle patterns for flap creation after small incision lenticule extraction. J Refract Surg. 2013;29:236-44.

5. Kling S, Spiru B, Hafezi F, et al. Biomechanical weakening of different retreatment options after small incision lenticule extraction (SMILE). J Refract Surg. 2017;33:193-8.
6. Chansue E, Tanehsakdi M, Swasdibutra S, et al. Safety and efficacy of VisuMax® circle patterns for flap creation and enhancement following small incision lenticule extraction. Eye Vis (Lond). 2015;2:21.
7. Donate D, Thaëron R. Preliminary evidence of successful enhancement after a primary SMILE procedure with the sub-cap-lenticule-extraction technique. J Refract Surg. 2015;31:708-10.
8. Titiyal JS, Kaur M, Rathi A, et al. Learning curve of small incision lenticule extraction: challenges & complications. Cornea. 2017 Aug 9. [Epub ahead of print]
9. Luft N, Ring MH, Dirisamer M, et al. Corneal epithelial remodeling induced by small incision lenticule extraction (SMILE). Invest Ophthalmol Vis Sci. 2016;57:176-83.
10. Netto MV, Mohan RR, Ambrósio R Jr, et al. Wound healing in the cornea: a review of refractive surgery complications and new prospects for therapy. Cornea. 2005;24:509-22.
11. Hersh PS, Schein OD, Steinert R. Characteristics influencing outcomes of excimer laser photorefractive keratectomy. Ophthalmology. 1996;103:1962-9.
12. Ivarsen A, Hjortdal JØ. Topography-guided photorefractive keratectomy for irregular astigmatism after small incision lenticule extraction. J Refract Surg. 2014;30:429-32.
13. Zhao J, Yao P, Chen Z, et al. Enhancement of femtosecond lenticule extraction for visual symptomatic eye after myopia correction. BMC Ophthalmol. 2014;14:68.

Chapter 11

SMILE versus Femtosecond LASIK: Weighing the Pros and Cons

Anubha Rathi, Manpreet Kaur, Anand Singh Brar, Ramkishor Sah, Jeewan S Titiyal

INTRODUCTION

The introduction of femtosecond (FS) laser technology to make lamellar corneal flaps in 2001 heralded a major change in the field of refractive surgery. Femtosecond laser-assisted in situ keratomileusis (FS-LASIK) has proven to be a safe, effective, and predictable procedure with consistent results and patient satisfaction. Since then, we have progressed from flap-based excimer laser ablation to FS-laser-assisted intrastromal refractive lenticule extraction. The flapless refractive lenticule extraction (ReLEx) using the technique of small incision lenticule extraction (SMILE) has recently gained popularity for the treatment of myopia and myopic astigmatism, but LASIK still remains the most commonly performed refractive surgery worldwide.

Till date, both FS-LASIK and SMILE have proven their efficacy, accuracy, and functional outcomes in their own domains. In this chapter, we have evaluated the advantages and disadvantages of both surgeries with respect to the surgical technique, refractive and physiological outcomes as well as complications.

HOW SMILE DIFFERS FROM LASIK?

The technique of ReLEx was initially reported in 2008 by Sekundo et al.; however, it received Food and Drug Administration (FDA) approval for the correction of myopia and myopic astigmatism recently in 2016.[1] SMILE is still in the developmental stages and the refractive applications of this novel procedure are continually expanding. There are numerous reports in literature proving its efficacy and accuracy, which reflect its rising popularity. Several recent studies have concluded that this flapless refractive surgery has good predictability, efficacy, and safety very similar to that of FS-LASIK.[1-4]

Though both procedures employ FS laser, they differ in terms of the surgical principle, technique, patient selection criteria as well as the postoperative outcomes.

SURGICAL PROCEDURE

Femtosecond-LASIK and SMILE differ in terms of basic surgical principle, laser parameters, and planning as well as the technique (Table 11.1).

- *Basic surgical principle*: Femtosecond-LASIK utilizes both FS laser and excimer laser for refractive correction. FS laser has a wavelength of

Table 11.1: Comparison of technical specifications, surgical technique, and case selection between small incision lenticule extraction (SMILE) and laser-assisted in situ keratomileusis (LASIK)

Parameter	*SMILE*	*LASIK*
Laser	Femtosecond laser	Femtosecond and excimer laser
IOP rise during docking	30–80 mm Hg	80–100 mm Hg
Risk of decentration	Lesser	Higher
FDA approved range of refractive error	Myopia from −1.00 D to −8.00 D with ≤−0.50 D cylinder MRSE of −8.25 D	Myopia up to −12 D, Astigmatism up to 6 D Hyperopia up to +6 D
Technique	Flapless refractive lenticule extraction	Flap-based excimer laser ablation
Treatment parameters	▪ Cap thickness 100–160 µm ▪ Cap diameter 6–9.6 mm ▪ Incision position 0–359° ▪ Incision width 2–5 mm ▪ Lenticule diameter 5–8 mm ▪ Transition zone 0.10 for CYL, 0 for SPH ▪ Minimum lenticule thickness 10–30 µm ▪ Lenticule side-cut angle 90–135°	▪ OZ: 6.5 mm for SPH 6.0 mm for CYL ▪ AZ: 7.1 mm for SPH 8.5 mm for CYL ▪ FD: 8.5 mm for SPH 8.7 mm for CYL
Patient selection	▪ Age ≥22 years ▪ Stable refractive error for past 1 year ▪ Off contact lenses ▪ Regular normal topography ▪ Adequate pachymetry ideally >500 µm ▪ RSBT >250 µm ▪ Active contact sports	▪ Age >18 years ▪ Stable refractive error for past 1 year ▪ Off contact lenses ▪ Regular normal topography ▪ Adequate pachymetry ideally >500 µm ▪ RSBT >280 µm ▪ Contraindicated in active contact sports: risk of flap dislodgement

(IOP: Intraocular pressure; FDA: Food and Drug Administration; MRSE: Manifest refraction spherical equivalent; CYL: Cylinder powers; SPH: Spherical powers; RSBT: Residual stromal bed thickness; OZ: Optical zone diameter; AZ: Ablation zone diameter; FD: Flap diameter).

1,053 nm that lies in the infrared range and its mechanism of action is based on the principle of photodisruption or photoionization. The FS laser is used to create a flap during LASIK, followed by excimer laser ablation for refractive correction. Conventionally used excimer laser is a 193 nm argon fluoride (ArF) laser and is based on the principle of photoablation. This involves breaking of covalent bonds between molecules. FS-LASIK machines have two separate workstations for FS and excimer laser, hence requiring the patient bed to be moved during the surgery from one station to the other.

SMILE is a purely FS laser-based procedure and utilizes a single, less cumbersome workstation. As there is no use of excimer laser, there is no odor of the burnt tissue as well, which is very apparent during FS-LASIK. Initial machines utilized FS laser with 200 kHz repetition rates for creating the intrastromal lenticule, while in the recent times, second generation 500 kHz FS laser devices have been developed. The VisuMax FS laser system (Carl Zeiss Meditec, Jena, Germany) produces ultrashort pulses of light of duration 220–580 fs with a pulse energy less than or equal to 300 nJ which are focused at a particular depth in the cornea.

- *Treatment parameters*: Treatment planning in SMILE has two components—a lenticule and a cap. Lenticule data is entered as per the refractive error to be corrected. The lenticule diameter can be in the range of 5–8 mm. The cap is kept 0.5–1 mm larger than the lenticule. The lenticule side cut angle is set at 90° and a 2–5 mm incision can be planned anywhere between 0° and 359°.

  The FS-LASIK on the other hand has the concept of an optical zone (OZ), ablation zone (AZ), and the flap diameter (FD). These three are closely related to each other and their dimensions depend on the refractive error and presence or absence of a cylinder power. For purely myopic spherical error, the authors prefer an OZ of 6.5 mm, AZ of 7.1 mm, and FD of 8.5 mm, while for coexistent astigmatism the OZ is decreased to 6 mm and the AZ and FD are increased to 8.5 mm and 8.7 mm, respectively. For hyperopic spherical errors, a smaller OZ with larger AZ and FD are chosen in FS-LASIK. The overlying cap thickness in SMILE and flap thickness in FS-LASIK can be altered as per the corneal pachymetry of the patient. The target refraction is entered as per the standard Burrato's LASIK nomogram.[5] Similar nomograms are in their budding phase for SMILE. While some surgeons extrapolate the flap-based lenticule extraction (FLEx) nomograms for SMILE as well, the authors prefer to use no correction factor for SMILE.
- *Docking*: The suction in case of SMILE is applied purely on the cornea unlike in FS-LASIK where it is also applied on adjacent sclera or conjunctiva. Hence there may be lesser incidence of subconjunctival hemorrhage post-docking. Also this ensures that intraocular pressure (IOP) rise

during this step is lesser as compared to FS-LASIK. SMILE creates a suction pressure of approximately 35 mm Hg and raises the IOP to only 30–80 mm Hg which allows the patient's vision and the intraocular circulation to be maintained during docking.[6] This allows the patient to visualize the green blinking light at the time of docking and produces better centration. FS-LASIK on the other hand generates suction at two levels, cornea and the limbus or sclera. This generates a higher pressure and IOP is seen to rise to as high as 100 mm Hg for few fractions of a second.[6] At this moment, the target light is not visible to the patient and there may be a risk of decentration leading to increased postoperative higher-order aberrations (HOAs). Also as the IOP rise is lesser during SMILE, it is speculated that the posterior segment pathologies secondary to the increased suction duration and pressure may be lesser post SMILE as compared to FS-LASIK.

- *Surgical Technique*: FS-LASIK involves FS laser-assisted creation of a corneal flap with around 110–120 μm thickness and lifting it, before ablating the residual bed with excimer laser. After docking, the FS laser cuts the flap of the preset diameter and thickness. The patient bed is then moved to the excimer workstation. The flap is gently lifted here and excimer laser ablation is completed after confirming the centration of the eye.

  The technique of SMILE demands greater expertise and surgical precision as it is purely lamellar and there is less room for maneuvering. The patient's eye is centered and docked with the curved interface cone before initiation of suction. The laser is then fired in the following order: the posterior cleavage plane defining the posterior surface of the refractive lenticule (spiral in), the lenticule side cut, the anterior cleavage plane defining the anterior surface of the refractive lenticule (spiral out) which exceeds the posterior plane by 0.5–1 mm and forms the anterior cap. Lastly the cap cut or incision is created. Till the entire sequence is over, laser foot pedal is continuously pressed. The docking and suction is then released. The cap cut or incision is finally opened to extract the already dissected lenticule as described in detail in Chapter 5 "Surgical Technique of Small Incision Lenticule Extraction".

PATIENT SELECTION CRITERIA

There is a certain degree of overlap in the patient selection criteria for both FS-LASIK and SMILE. There are few patients who may be more suited for one of the two procedures. Weighing the two options in totality is usually the rule.

Refractive Error

The FS-LASIK is approved for myopia up to –12 D, astigmatism up to 6 D and up to +6 D hyperopia. SMILE is FDA approved for myopia from –1.00 D to

–8.00 D with upto –0.50 D cylinder and manifest refraction spherical equivalent (MRSE) of –8.25 D, though it is currently being used off-label for a wider range of errors with proven efficacy. SMILE has recently also been used for hyperopia correction even though FDA approval for the same is still awaited. In case of very low refractive errors such as less than –2 DS, the expected thickness of the refractive lenticule may become too thin to discern intraoperatively and the lenticule may be too flimsy to handle. Such cases may be better candidates for FS-LASIK.

Patient Profile

A SMILE procedure costs the patient a little more than double the amount of FS-LASIK. Hence, the socioeconomic status and affordability of the patient itself sometimes makes it easy to choose between these two options and is an important factor in developing nations. Overanxious, hyperactive persons and those suffering from a known psychiatric illness should best be avoided for both SMILE and LASIK as outcome of any refractive surgery depends majorly on patient's cooperation. As for FS-LASIK, patients with history of viral keratitis, autoimmune diseases, severe dry eyes, uncontrolled diabetes, pregnancy or lactation should be avoided in case selection of SMILE as well. An ideal patient for both SMILE and LASIK is a patient with stable refractive error, not using contact lenses for at least 2 weeks with a normal topography scan, adequate pachymetry, and no other contraindication for the surgery.

There are a few cases where SMILE may be chosen over LASIK owing to its flapless nature. These are people actively involved in sports, especially contact sports and swimming, as the presence of a flap predisposes them to a higher risk of flap dislocation at any time after surgery. Some reports have revealed there is a lesser incidence of dry eye post-SMILE as compared to LASIK but nonetheless preexisting dry eye of any severity remains a contraindication for SMILE.

Corneal Topography

A regular corneal topography pattern with no features suggestive of ectasia is required before planning both SMILE and FS-LASIK. The criteria followed by the authors include maximum corneal power (Kmax) less than 47.2 D, posterior elevation less than +20 µm on Scheimpflug imaging and less than +40 µm on Placido's disk or slit scanning system, with normal Belin-Ambrosio enhanced ectasia map on Scheimpflug imaging. Any evidence of irregular astigmatism or forme fruste keratoconus is a contraindication for refractive surgery. This stands true both for SMILE and FS-LASIK. It has been speculated that SMILE may be associated with lesser risk of ectasia but in view of inconsistent results in this regard and a few reports of post-SMILE ectasia coming up, the current selection protocol is such that all possible borderline cases must be excluded at the outset.

Corneal Pachymetry and Residual Bed Thickness

Sekundo et al. in 2010 introduced SMILE for patients with the central corneal thickness more than 500 μm and the calculated residual stromal bed thickness (RSBT) after treatment more than 250 μm.[2] Safe limit for RSBT in FS-LASIK is usually 280–300 μm. Hence the difference is not very significant. The cap diameter in SMILE is kept around 110–120 μm quite similar to the flap in FS-LASIK. The amount of tissue removed or ablated per diopter in SMILE is calculated to be 13 μm versus 17 μm in FS-LASIK.[7] Hence the safety bracket is only slightly spaced apart in case of SMILE and offers no significant added advantage in this regard. Most of the surgeons do not prefer to tread into that difference zone anyhow. So the patient selection criteria in terms of pachymetry and RSBT overlap to a large extent for both SMILE and LASIK.

Contraindications

Absolute contraindications for SMILE and FS-LASIK are very similar and include uncooperative, anxious patient with known uncontrolled systemic disease, psychiatric illness, severe dry eyes, unstable refractive error, evidence of ectasia or irregular astigmatism on corneal topography map with thinner inadequate pachymetry.

OUTCOMES

SMILE is an alternative procedure to conventional FS-LASIK and is not proven till date to be consistently superior in any aspect. It has been postulated to be better in terms of maintained corneal biomechanics with decreased denervation, lesser incidence of dry eye, and no flap-related complications. There have been reports of smooth visual recovery with consistent, predictable, and effective refractive outcomes as well. This section predominantly highlights the differences in the outcome profile of SMILE and FS-LASIK (Table 11.2).

Corneal Biomechanics

The anterior stroma is stronger than the posterior stroma by almost 25%. The interlamellar proteoglycan bonding is responsible for the strength of central portion of the cornea while the peripheral and anterior strength depend on the pattern, arrangement, and interconnections between the stromal lamellae. Corneal biomechanics refers to the response of cornea to external forces applied and is summed up by the interaction between the externally applied force, the intrinsic corneal resistance factor (CRF) or corneal hysteresis (CH),

Table 11.2: Comparison of outcomes of small incision lenticule extraction (SMILE) and laser-assisted in situ keratomileusis (LASIK)

Parameter	SMILE	FS-LASIK
Corneal biomechanics	Better postoperative tensile strength	Lesser postoperative tensile strength
Refractive outcomes ▪ Predictability ▪ Efficacy ▪ Safety ▪ Stability	Equally predictable, efficacious, safe, and stable	Equally predictable, efficacious, safe, and stable
Visual recovery	Delayed visual recovery	No significant delay
Dry eye and ocular surface-related problems	▪ Healthier ocular surface ▪ Less incidence of dry eye	▪ More incidence of dry eye ▪ Increased tear film inflammatory mediators
Risk of ectasia	Less risk (inconsistent reports)	Slightly higher risk
Complications	▪ Intraoperative complications related to lenticule dissection and extraction ▪ No flap-related complications	Higher flap-related complications in early phase
Retreatment	▪ SMILE cannot be repeated ▪ Second stage flap-based procedure or PRK	Second stage repeat LASIK (relift original flap) or PRK
Learning curve	▪ More tedious ▪ Requires stepwise approach	Less tedious

(FS-LASIK: Femtosecond-laser-assisted in situ keratomileusis; PRK: Photorefractive keratectomy).

and the IOP. Ocular response analyzer (ORA) and Corvis ST (Corneal Visualization Scheimpflug Technology) have been used to evaluate corneal biomechanics, and various studies have revealed a significant reduction in CRF and CH after both LASIK and SMILE.[8,9] However, the decrease in biomechanical strength is significantly less after SMILE.

The superior biomechanical stability after SMILE may be attributed to the differential healing that occurs post-SMILE and leads to possible fibrous scarring at stromal lamellar level, thereby strengthening it. Other possible explanation is that LASIK flaps are usually larger while cap and lenticule diameters in SMILE are smaller; hence the stronger peripheral collagen bundles are saved in SMILE. The level of tissue removal or ablation differs in SMILE and LASIK. LASIK being more anterior weakens the anterior stroma which is responsible for corneal biomechanical strength (Figs. 11.1A and B).

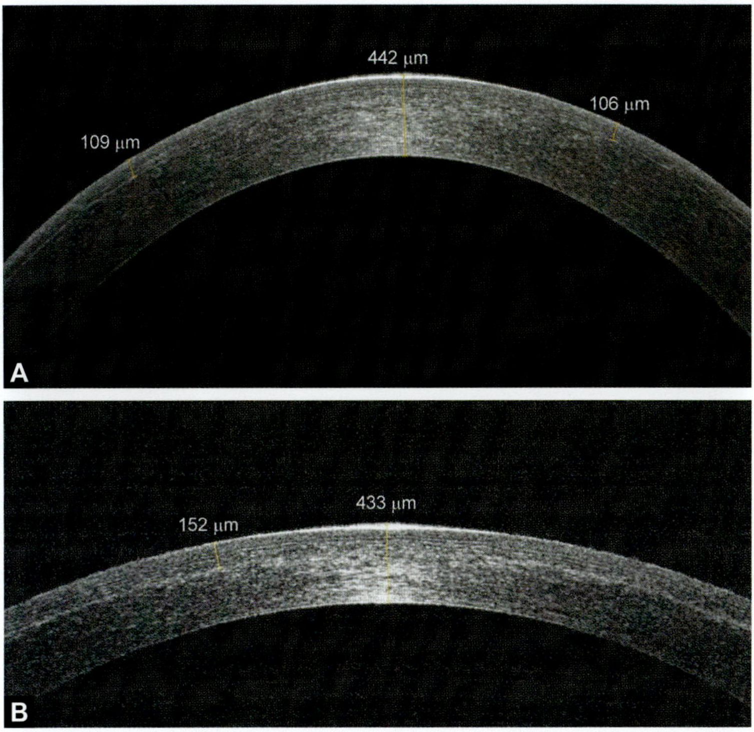

Figs. 11.1A and B: (A) One month postoperative laser-assisted in situ keratomileusis (LASIK) interface as imaged on anterior segment optical coherence tomography (ASOCT), with a thin flap. (B) One month postoperative small incision lenticule extraction (SMILE) interface as imaged on ASOCT. The anterior stromal fibers are relatively well-preserved due to an increased depth of cap.

Reinstein et al. estimated the stromal tensile strength after photorefractive keratectomy (PRK), LASIK, and SMILE and revealed that the postoperative tensile strength after SMILE was around 25% higher than LASIK and 10% more than PRK.[10]

Corneal Innervation and Ocular Surface Stability

The damage to sub-basal nerve plexus is responsible for the dry eye syndrome post-refractive surgery. As SMILE is essentially flapless, the corneal nerves are salvaged and hence dry eye and related complications are lesser as compared to LASIK. In vivo confocal microscopy has been used to assess the sub-basal nerve plexus after refractive surgery, and the reduction in length and density is more in LASIK than SMILE (Figs. 11.2A to F).[11,12]

The corneal nerve regeneration is faster after SMILE, though the nerve recovery patterns are similar in both LASIK and SMILE after 6 months.[12]

The central corneal sensitivity is relatively preserved after SMILE, which may explain the decreased incidence of dry eyes.[11,12] Denoyer et al. evaluated

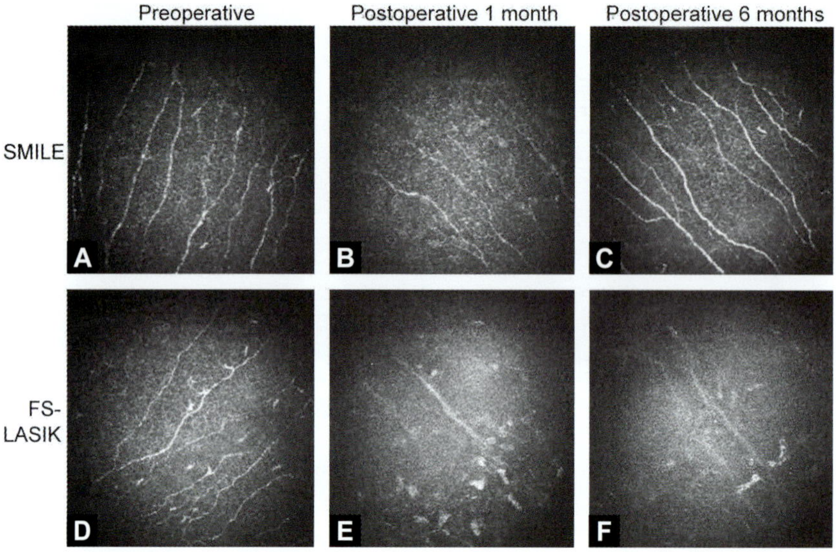

Figs. 11.2A to F: Sub-basal nerve fiber layer on confocal microscopy. (A) Preoperative sub-basal nerve fiber layer before small incision lenticule extraction (SMILE); (B) Sub-basal nerve fiber layer 1 month after SMILE; (C) Sub-basal nerve fiber layer 6 months after SMILE; (D) Preoperative sub-basal nerve fiber layer before LASIK; (E) Sub-basal nerve fiber layer 1 month after LASIK; (F) Sub-basal nerve fiber layer 6 months after LASIK.

the indices of dry eye disease post-FS-LASIK and SMILE. Ocular surface disease index, tear film breakup time, tear osmolarity, and dry eye severity scores were better in post-SMILE cases as compared to LASIK.[13] Gao et al. in 2014 studied the role of tear inflammatory mediators in ocular surface rehabilitation post-SMILE and FS-LASIK. It was revealed that interleukin-6 (IL-6) and nerve growth factor (NGF) levels correlated with ocular surface changes in SMILE and LASIK.[14] A meta-analysis comparing dry eye disease after SMILE and LASIK observed the occurrence of transient dry eyes after both procedures, with milder subjective symptoms after SMILE.[15]

Refractive Outcomes

Recent literature suggests that SMILE demonstrates reasonable predictability, safety, stability, and efficacy, similar to that of FS-LASIK.[11,16]

- *Visual recovery*: Most studies suggest that though the restoration of objective refraction post-SMILE is as early as in LASIK, the visual acuity may show delayed recovery. This may be attributed to the microscopic irregularities induced in the stroma at the time of dissection. These irregularities have decreased now with the second generation machines with 500 kHz repetition rates. Agca et al. observed that the interface reflectivity of the corneas that underwent SMILE was significantly more in the initial 3 months post-surgery as compared to LASIK-treated eyes.[9]

This higher reflectivity is possibly due to activation of keratocytes in SMILE and could be indicative of delayed visual recovery.

- *Visual acuity—predictability, efficacy, safety, and stability*: SMILE is comparable to FS-LASIK in terms of predictability, efficacy, safety, and stability of the refractive outcomes. Few studies have also demonstrated the superiority of SMILE over FS-LASIK in terms of the visual acuity parameters.[11,16] Predictability of a refractive procedure refers to the extent to which the attempted spherical equivalent correction is obtained after the procedure. Kamiya et al. observed that 100% of eyes that underwent SMILE were within ±0.5 D and ±1 D at 1-year follow-up.[17] The predictability of LASIK is estimated to be between 78.2% and 96.7% in published studies.[18]

  Stability of the outcome is very important for patient satisfaction. Regression rates in SMILE have not been extensively reported in literature as long-term follow-up studies for the same are lacking. However, SMILE is associated with less postoperative epithelial remodeling as well as a less exuberant stromal healing response, and has been postulated to have a decreased incidence of regression as compared to LASIK. The enhancement rates reported after SMILE are much lower than those observed after FS-LASIK.

  Blum et al. observed 41 eyes after FLEx for 5 years.[17] The mean annual regression during this period was noted to be –0.07 D, which is comparable to the annual regression rate of –0.12 D after 15 years of follow-up post-LASIK.[19]

- *Visual quality*: SMILE induces less HOAs than conventional FS-LASIK. It also reduces the induction of spherical aberrations as compared to LASIK. However, SMILE has been observed to induce more horizontal and vertical coma compared with wavefront-guided LASIK, indicating a less precise centration of SMILE procedure.[20,21] The contrast sensitivity after SMILE and LASIK is similar, with a mild decrease observed after both procedures.[11,16]

LEARNING CURVE

SMILE is an intrastromal procedure that is not affected by the external parameters such as temperature and humidity. However, the intrastromal manipulations may be technically challenging for a novice surgeon, in contrast to flap-based procedures which can be mastered with relative ease. A steep learning curve is associated with SMILE, and the procedure requires finesse and precision. Various intraoperative complications may be experienced by the surgeon during the initial few cases of SMILE. Lenticule identification and dissection is particularly challenging for a beginner, and intraoperative difficulties may result in suboptimal visual outcomes. Hence a stepwise approach is recommended before jumping on to SMILE for the first time.

COMPLICATIONS

Both FS-LASIK and SMILE are associated with their own set of complications. These complications may be higher in the initial learning phase, especially with SMILE. Intraoperative complications of LASIK are usually related to the creation of flap, such as flap tears, buttonholing, free cap, and free flap. These flap-related complications have further reduced with the advent of FS laser technology, and the shift from microkeratome to FS-laser flaps.

SMILE does not entail any flap-related complications; however, it is associated with unique complications mainly related to lenticule handling and extraction. Difficult lenticule extraction, intraoperative suction loss, tearing of lenticule, and side-cut extension have all been reported during SMILE.[22]

Postoperative complications common to both SMILE and LASIK include overtreatment, undertreatment, regression, and epithelial erosions. SMILE is associated with greater biomechanical stability as compared to LASIK and has a lower risk of ectasia. The reported incidence of post-LASIK ectasia lies between 0.06% and 0.8%.[23] In contrast, only few isolated cases of post-SMILE ectasia have been reported.

ENHANCEMENTS AND RETREATMENT

A repeat SMILE procedure for postoperative enhancement or retreatment is generally not feasible, owing to the risk of creating multiple dissection planes. Secondary procedures after an initial SMILE involves the use of excimer laser ablation in the form of either PRK, thin-flap LASIK or circle pattern of VisuMax laser to convert the cap into a flap. The retreatment options are associated with a loss of the biomechanical advantages of SMILE. Moreover, this means that a SMILE refractive suite is not self-sufficient, and always requires a standby excimer laser system.

In contrast, post-LASIK enhancement is technically easy, and requires a simple relifting of the flap followed by excimer laser ablation, or a surface ablation.

Retreatment results after both LASIK and SMILE have been favorable. It is advisable to wait for refractive stability before planning a retreatment in both the cases.

WEIGHING THE PROS AND CONS

Even with the advent of SMILE, FS-LASIK still continues to hold its fort. This indicates that though both the surgeries have their own pros and cons; they are here to stay! Weighing the pros and cons depending on the patient

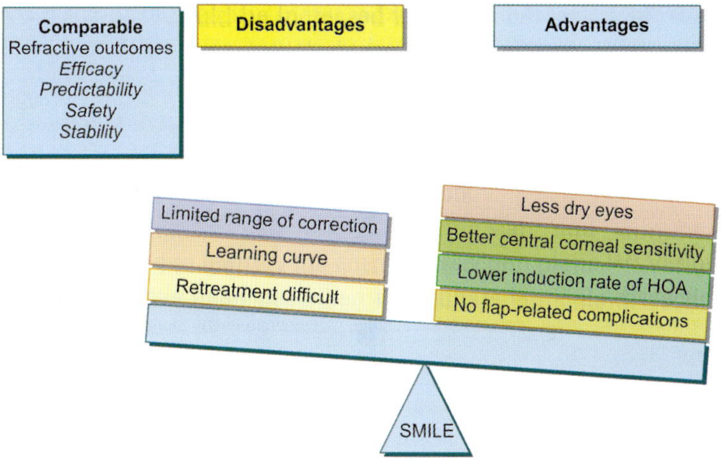

Fig. 11.3: Weighing the pros and cons of small incision lenticule extraction (SMILE) and laser-assisted in situ keratomileusis (LASIK).
(HOA: Higher-order aberration).

profile, surgeon expertise, amount of refractive error, corneal topography, and pachymetry is of utmost importance (Fig. 11.3).

CONCLUSION

Small incision lenticule extraction has proven to be equally efficacious, predictable, and safe as compared to FS-LASIK. At the same time, it preserves the biomechanical integrity of the cornea and is associated with lesser incidence of dry eye. Long-term follow-up of SMILE is still awaited to conclusively prove its efficacy. It offers a significant learning curve to surgeons but is a promising technique once mastered.

REFERENCES

1. Sekundo W, Kunert K, Russmann C, et al. First efficacy and safety study of femtosecond lenticule extraction for the correction of myopia: six-month results. J Cataract Refract Surg. 2008;34(9):1513-20.
2. Sekundo W, Kunert KS, Blum M. Small incision corneal refractive surgery using the small incision lenticule extraction (SMILE) procedure for the correction of myopia and myopic astigmatism: results of a 6-month prospective study. Br J Ophthalmol. 2011;95(3):335-9.
3. Shah R, Shah S, Sengupta S. Results of small incision lenticule extraction: all-in-one femtosecond laser refractive surgery. J Cataract Refract Surg. 2011;37(1):127-37.
4. Vestergaard A, Ivarsen A, Asp S, et al. Femtosecond (FS) laser vision correction procedure for moderate to high myopia: a prospective study of ReLEx flex, and comparison with a retrospective study of FS-laser in situ keratomileusis. Acta Ophthalmol. 2013;91(4):355-62.
5. Buratto L, Ferrari M, Genisi C. Myopic keratomileusis with the excimer laser: one-year follow-up. Refract Corneal Surg. 1993;9(1):12-9.

6. Vetter JM, Holzer MP, Teping C, et al. Intraocular pressure during corneal flap preparation: comparison among four femtosecond lasers in porcine eyes. J Refract Surg. 2011;27(6):427-33.
7. Ganesh S, Brar S. Clinical outcomes of small incision lenticule extraction with accelerated cross-linking (ReLEx SMILE Xtra) in patients with thin corneas and borderline topography. J Ophthalmol. 2015;2015:263412.
8. Frings A, Linke SJ, Baeur EL, et al. Effects of laser in situ keratomileusis (LASIK) on corneal biomechanical measurements with the Corvis ST tonometer. Clin Ophthalmol. 2015;9:305-11.
9. Agca A, Ozgurhan EB, Demirok A, et al. Comparison of corneal hysteresis and corneal resistance factor after small incision lenticule extraction and femtosecond laser-assisted LASIK: a prospective fellow eye study. Cont Lens Anterior Eye. 2014;37(2):77-80.
10. Reinstein DZ, Archer TJ, Gobbe M. Small incision lenticule extraction (SMILE) history, fundamentals of a new refractive surgery technique and clinical outcomes. Eye Vis (Lond). 2014;1:3.
11. Zhang Y, Shen Q, Jia Y, et al. Clinical outcomes of SMILE and FS-LASIK used to treat myopia: a meta-analysis. J Refract Surg. 2016;32(4):256-65.
12. Li M, Niu L, Qin B, et al. Confocal comparison of corneal reinnervation after small incision lenticule extraction (SMILE) and femtosecond laser in situ keratomileusis (FS-LASIK). PLoS One. 2013;8(12):e81435.
13. Denoyer A, Landman E, Trinh L, et al. Dry eye disease after refractive surgery: comparative outcomes of small incision lenticule extraction versus LASIK. Ophthalmology. 2015;122(4):669-76.
14. Gao S, Li S, Liu L, et al. Early changes in ocular surface and tear inflammatory mediators after small-incision lenticule extraction and femtosecond laser-assisted laser in situ keratomileusis. PLoS One. 2014;9(9):e107370.
15. Shen Z, Zhu Y, Song X, et al. Dry eye after small incision lenticule extraction (SMILE) versus femtosecond laser-assisted in situ keratomileusis (FS-LASIK) for myopia: a meta-analysis. PLoS One. 2016;11(12):e0168081.
16. Shen Z, Shi K, Yu Y, et al. Small incision lenticule extraction (SMILE) versus femtosecond laser-assisted in situ keratomileusis (FS-LASIK) for myopia: a systematic review and meta-analysis. PLoS One. 2016;11(7):e0158176.
17. Kamiya K, Shimizu K, Igarashi A, et al. Comparison of visual acuity, higher-order aberrations and corneal asphericity after refractive lenticule extraction and wavefront-guided laser-assisted in situ keratomileusis for myopia. Br J Ophthalmol. 2013;97(8):968-75.
18. Shah R, Shah S, Sengupta S. Results of small incision lenticule extraction: all-in-one femtosecond laser refractive surgery. J Cataract Refract Surg. 2011;37(1): 127-37.
19. Blum M, Flach A, Kunert KS, et al. Five-year results of refractive lenticule extraction. J Cataract Refract Surg. 2014;40(9):1425-9.
20. Ye M, Liu C, Liao R, et al. SMILE and wavefront-guided LASIK out-compete other refractive surgeries in ameliorating the induction of high-order aberrations in anterior corneal surface. J Ophthalmol. 2016;2016:8702162.
21. Chen X, Wang Y, Zhang J, et al. Comparison of ocular higher-order aberrations after SMILE and wavefront-guided femtosecond LASIK for myopia. BMC Ophthalmol. 2017;17(1):42.
22. Titiyal JS, Kaur M, Rathi A, et al. Learning curve of small incision lenticule extraction: challenges & complications. Cornea. 2017 Aug 9. [Epub ahead of print].
23. Binder PS. Analysis of ectasia after laser in situ keratomileusis: risk factors. J Cataract Refract Surg. 2007;33(9):1530-8.

Chapter

12

Future Technological Advances in Small Incision Lenticule Extraction

Harathy Selvan, Manpreet Kaur, Jeewan S Titiyal

INTRODUCTION

The VisuMax femtosecond laser-assisted small incision lenticule extraction (SMILE) received the Food and Drug Administration (FDA) approval in 2016 for the correction of myopia and myopic astigmatism. However, the applications of this evolving procedure cannot be contained under the above limits. The safety and efficacy of SMILE in a wider range of myopia and astigmatism, as well as hyperopia is under evaluation. The refractive lenticule obtained after SMILE has the potential to be used in various tissue additive surgeries for stromal expansion and in the management of corneal ectatic disorders. Moreover, the combination of SMILE with collagen cross-linking (CXL) may open new avenues in the refractive correction and biomechanical stabilization of corneas at risk for ectasia. The diverse applications of SMILE, present and future, are explained in this chapter.

EXPANDING REFRACTIVE APPLICATIONS OF SMILE

Myopia

At present, SMILE is approved for use in cases of myopia with manifest refraction spherical equivalent (MRSE) of less than or equal to –8.25 D, which may include a sphere ranging from –1 DS to –8 DS, and astigmatism of less than or equal to –0.5 DC. FDA phase 2 trials are being conducted to evaluate the safety and efficacy of SMILE in patients with spherical myopia of –1 D to –10 D, astigmatism of –0.75 D to –3 D and MRSE of –11.50 D or less.[1]

Hyperopia

Surgical correction of hyperopia has always been an extra mile beyond the traditional refractive expertise. This is in part due to the challenge in steepening the central cornea, unpredictability of the refractive outcomes and a higher risk of regression. The nomogram for hyperopic SMILE is still evolving.

The lenticule profile in hyperopia is significantly different from myopia, as explained in Table 12.1.[2] The peculiarities of hyperopic lenticules are that they are thinnest at the center, thicker at the periphery, and incorporate an additional large mid-peripheral transition zone (approximately 2 mm) and a smaller clearance zone (Fig. 12.1). This is in contrast to the myopic SMILE lenticule, where the central region is the thickest and the transition zone ranges from 0 mm to 0.1 mm, depending upon the presence of astigmatism. Briefly, the pattern of lenticule creation in hyperopia is spiral-in for the posterior surface cut and spiral-out for rest of the components—transition zone, lenticule border, anterior surface and side cut, in that same order.[2] The femtosecond laser delivery for hyperopic lenticule creation takes 4–6 seconds more than in myopia, due to the delay in the creation of a large transition zone.[2,3] This may result in higher stromal collagen lamellar distortion and lead to delayed postoperative visual recovery. A modification in the treatment protocol has been proposed that will allow the simultaneous creation of posterior lenticule interface as well as the transition zone in a spiral-in manner.

Significant postoperative regression is still observed, with only 22% of patients within 0.5 D of the intended correction and 78% of eyes within 1.00 D of target refraction at the end of 9 months.[2] Various methods are being suggested to improve the refractive predictability and stability. A modified

Table 12.1: Differences between myopic and hyperopic SMILE lenticule

Variable	*Myopic lenticule*	*Hyperopic lenticule*
Lenticule characteristics		
Center	Thickest	Thinnest
Periphery	Thinner than center	Thicker than center
Transition zone	0 mm in sphere 0.1 mm in cylinder	Large (2 mm) Between optical and clearance zone
Clearance zone	Larger	Relatively smaller
Lenticule creation sequence and time		
Sequence of events during creation	Posterior surface → lenticule border → anterior surface → cap incision	Posterior surface → transition zone → lenticule border → anterior surface → cap incision
Time for lenticule creation	25–28 seconds (30–35 seconds in old software)	+4–6 seconds more than myopia
Pattern of creation		
Posterior surface	Spiral in	Spiral in
Transition zone	Spiral out	Spiral out
Anterior surface	Spiral out	Spiral out

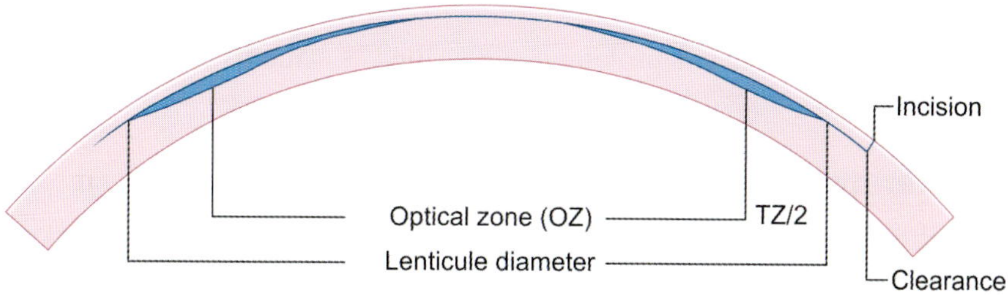

Fig. 12.1: Hyperopic lenticule.
(TZ: Transition zone).

nomogram that aims for primary overcorrection by 0.75 D may help counter the long-term regression, which is approximately 0.5 D in magnitude. Moreover, it has been observed that improving the lenticule profile by making a larger optical and transition zone may reduce the amount of postoperative regression.[2] Compensatory epithelial thickening is a major factor responsible for regression in post-SMILE hyperopia.[2,3] The large optical and transition zones lead to a reduced curvature gradient in the region of maximum tissue removal, thereby reducing the compensatory epithelial thickening in this region and the subsequent risk of regression. The mean optical zone diameter of hyperopic SMILE is larger than the mean optical zone diameter of hyperopic laser-assisted in situ keratomileusis (LASIK), with a similar induction of spherical aberrations.[4]

Myopic Astigmatism

Treatment of patients with myopic astigmatism has revealed that though acceptable correction of spherical equivalent can be achieved, astigmatic undercorrection may occur. The magnitude of undercorrection may be as high as 13% per diopter in cases of low astigmatism (<2.5 D) and 16% per diopter of attempted correction in high astigmatism (≥2.5 D) respectively. Also, a mild torsion of the cylinder axis can occur in cases of low astigmatism.[5] An astigmatism of up to three diopters does not hinder the predictability of postoperative outcomes, in contrast to patients with higher cylinders, who exhibit greater risks for re-treatment.[6]

Presbyopia

A new technique called the "**P**r**E**sbyopic **A**llogenic **R**efractive **L**enticule" (PEARL) inlay has been described, where an allograft SMILE lenticule is used to treat presbyopia.[7] A button of 1 mm is trephined from the central part of the lenticule to obtain a ring of lenticule. A femtosecond laser pocket is created at around the depth of 120 μm, and the inlay is implanted in the nondominant eye. This procedure produced spectacle independence for near, intermediate and distant activities. It has been proven to be safe and efficacious; however, long-term results are not known at present. The presbyopic corneal inlay led to a prolateness of cornea as evidenced in the corneal topography of operated eyes.[7]

Postkeratoplasty Refractive Correction

Refractive lenticule extraction in postkeratoplasty eyes may be undertaken as soon as 3 months after complete suture removal.[8,9] It has the advantage of tackling both myopia and myopic astigmatism in a single stage, in contrast to the traditional incisional procedures employed in postkeratoplasty refractive error management. Minor modifications are required in the existing technique, such as the usage of a small suction cup, and setting the lenticule diameter smaller than the graft size. The results of this procedure have been encouraging. It is a highly efficacious and safe procedure with resultant uncorrected visual acuity equivalent to 90% of the patient's previous best-corrected visual acuity (BCVA). There is no added disadvantage to the graft-host junction or the donor endothelium. However, the risk of undercorrection exists, due to cyclotorsion, lenticule decentration, eccentric grafts, change in graft tension, resistance along fibrous suture tracks, inappropriate laser settings and postoperative epithelial hyperplasia. Nevertheless, it confers stability with moderate accuracy and promotes early visual rehabilitation.[8]

Myopia with Corneal Opacity

Traditionally, a clear cornea is preferred for laser refractive procedures. This is partly attributed to the unpredictable penetration and scanning by femtolaser as well as difficult flap lifting in scarred corneas. In such cases, irrespective of the location of the scars, SMILE remains a viable option since corneal opacities of density value 20.4–85.8 are penetrable by the VisuMax system.[10] However, the corneal opacity tends to persist even after surgery, and hence this procedure should be preferred in cases with non-central involving scars.

COMBINED SMILE AND COLLAGEN CROSS-LINKING

Collagen cross-linking is an established treatment modality to halt the progression of ectasia and provide refractive stability in eyes with progressive keratoconus. Refractive surgical procedures such as LASIK and photorefractive keratectomy (PRK) have been combined with CXL to prevent ectasia in thin corneas with high magnitude of refractive errors.

The preservation of anterior stroma and the absence of a flap in SMILE have been observed to confer greater biomechanical stability as compared to LASIK. The potential of SMILE combined with simultaneous CXL is currently being evaluated for refractive correction in cases at high-risk of ectasia or with evident forme fruste keratoconus. The combined procedure will serve the dual purpose of correcting the refractive error as well as strengthening the at-risk cornea.

SMILE combined with accelerated CXL (SMILE Xtra) has been tried in cases that are at moderate- to high-risk of ectasia as per the Randleman ectasia scoring system. SMILE Xtra has also been evaluated in cases at low-risk for ectasia, but with coexistent family history of keratoconus or history of atopy.

The role of SMILE combined with conventional CXL has been investigated in cases with early keratoconus (grade I and II, Amsler-Krumeich grading system).

The procedure involves intrastromal application of riboflavin after extracting the refractive lenticule as per the described surgical technique. The protocols vary for accelerated and conventional CXL. SMILE Xtra involves the application of 0.22–0.25% of riboflavin in saline (VibeX Xtra, Avedro) for a total duration of 45–60 seconds, followed by application of ultraviolet (UV) light.[11,12] The total energy used in SMILE Xtra ranged from 0.8 J/cm^2 to 3.4 J/cm^2 as per different protocols.[11,12] Ng et al. employed UV-A irradiation of 18 mW/cm^2 for 45 seconds (total energy: 0.8 J/cm^2), and Ganesh et al. employed irradiation of 45 mW/cm^2 for 75 seconds (total energy: 3.4 J/cm^2).[11,12]

The Aztec protocol has been recommended by the investigators in cases with early keratoconus undergoing SMILE with CXL. It involves the intrastromal application of 0.1% riboflavin in 20% dextran every 1–3 minutes for a total duration of 15 minutes, following which UV-A irradiation (370 nm, 3 mW/cm^2) is given for 30 minutes to achieve total energy application of 5.4 J/cm^2.[13] The riboflavin application is continued during UV irradiation.

Favorable visual outcomes have been reported in cases of SMILE combined with CXL, with 73% of eyes achieving refractive outcomes within 0.5 D, and 100% achieving refractive outcomes within 1 D of emmetropia. However, significant postoperative haze was present in all cases, though it spontaneously resolved by 3 months. Progression of keratoconus was not observed in the follow-up ranging from 1 to 2 years.

SMILE Xtra employed lower total energy of 0.8–3.4 J/cm^2. The incidence of significant postoperative haze was less and no case developed ectasia. Predictable refractive outcomes were achieved; however, an undercorrection was observed at 6 months with only 67% of eyes achieving an uncorrected distance visual acuity (UDVA) of 20/20 in one study.

SMILE with CXL is emerging as a promising technique for high-risk cases for ectasia or cases with pre-existing mild ectasia. It provides spectacle-independence along with strengthening the cornea. The potential may be limited by the development of postoperative haze; however, the success of accelerated

CXL with lower total energies may help achieve optimal outcomes. Further investigations are needed to help establish a uniform protocol that maximizes the biomechanical benefits without compromising on the quality of vision.

SMILE FOR RE-TREATMENT AFTER REFRACTIVE SURGERY

Conventionally, a re-treatment after SMILE is considered challenging as SMILE cannot be repeated. The risk of creating multiple interfaces limits the potential of SMILE to be used as an effective re-treatment option after SMILE. However, recent innovative techniques have employed SMILE as a re-treatment option after an initial LASIK or SMILE procedure.

SMILE in Thick-Flap LASIK

In cases of operated LASIK, the residual stromal bed is pristine and responsible for the corneal biomechanical strength henceforth. So, it is vital to maintain its integrity to avoid future inadvertent complications. At the same time, the flap tissue practically has nil contribution to the corneal strength, and hence, can be exploited in cases requiring re-treatment. SMILE can be the rescue resort in such situations, especially when the stromal bed is thin and the flap is thick, wherein the new refractive lenticule can be created in the flap itself. Satisfactory visual and anatomical outcomes were achieved after this procedure was undertaken in a case.[14]

Repeat SMILE

Till recently, a repeat SMILE was not considered feasible. However, femtosecond laser may be used to create only the second lenticule cut and lenticule side-cut, with respect to the original interface and incisions. Utilizing the old and the new cuts, the re-treatment is possible either anterior to the original interface (in-the-cap-SMILE) or beneath the original interface (sub-cap-lenticule extraction).[15-17]

However, the procedure is not validated as yet, and further technological advancements may help in the development of precise nomograms and softwares to enable a repeat SMILE procedure.

APPLICATIONS OF REFRACTIVE LENTICULE OF SMILE

The refractive lenticule extracted in SMILE may have diverse potential applications in various tissue additive procedures. It may be used as an onlay or an inlay, either in the same patient or as an allograft in different patients. Currently, research is ongoing to explore the myriad applications of the stromal tissue, and it may herald the development of promising future techniques for management of various ocular pathologies.

Femtosecond laser intrastromal lenticular implantation (FILI) has been developed, which incorporates the creation of a femtolaser-assisted intrastromal pocket followed by the insertion of previously harvested SMILE lenticule. The technique is based on Barraquer's law of thickness which states that cornea is steepened by intrastromal lenticule insertion of known thickness and power into a femtolaser created pocket.[18] The SMILE lenticule thus implanted may either be extracted from the same patient (autograft) or a different patient (allograft).

Autograft

A tissue is referred to as an autograft, when it facilitates autologous implantation. In the setting of refractive surgery, an autograft lenticule may either be implanted in the same eye at a later date or the contralateral eye at the same sitting. The latter situation occurs when patients have myopia in one eye and hyperopia in the other eye. The myopic eye can be treated with SMILE, and the lenticule extracted can be used as an autograft for the other eye. A recent study evaluating this technique showed it to be safe and effective. The lenticule was well-located, uniform and transparent.[19]

The SMILE lenticule may be cryopreserved and reimplanted in the same patient at a later date. A reimplantation may be required to restore the lost stromal volume in cases of unexpected postsurgical ectasia, followed by CXL to arrest progression. Similarly, reimplantation may also be desired in cases of presbyopia, where it can aid in creating monovision.[20]

Allograft

An allograft refers to a tissue that is harvested from a genetically unlike donor of the same species.

Treatment of Hyperopia

A refractive lenticule extracted from a myopic patient may be used for correction of hyperopia in another patient. The lenticule can be stored in donor corneal culture media or cryopreserved before use. This procedure is termed "endokeratophakia" when undertaken in aphakic patients.[21]

Though these augmentation procedures appear self-contained, they are still in their initial stages and need further refinement. The refractive outcomes after lenticule implantation in aphakia have not been satisfactory.

Tectonic Keratoplasty with Femtosecond Laser Intrastromal Lenticule

Tectonic keratoplasty with femtosecond laser intrastromal lenticule (TEKIL) is a novel procedure wherein the SMILE lenticule is used to provide anatomic support to maintain globe integrity in cases of large corneal ulcers with impending perforations or frank corneal perforations. It has been used as an emergency measure and resulted in significant improvement in BCVA at the final follow-up along with anatomic success in all cases. This procedure may be repeated several times as a temporary measure, with more than one lenticule piece per procedure, thus improving conditions for the final optical procedures.[22] The lenticules may also be stored stacked up one over the other (up to four have been reported) and used later.[23] The greatest advantage of this procedure lies in the absence of any reports of rejection or perforation till date. They can also be augmented with amniotic membrane grafts.

Corneal Stromal Equivalents

While TEKIL is the direct application of the refractive lenticule to provide tectonic support, stromal equivalents are processed lenticules which in addition to aiding the globe integrity, also repair the anterior corneal stromal damage and promote reorganization and transparency after deep corneal defects and perforations. In view of inadequate lenticule thickness and turgor, and the risk of realignment on using multiple individual lenticules, the innovation of corneal stromal equivalent (CSE) was sought. Refractive lenticules measuring 6.6 mm in diameter and central thickness greater than or equal to 100 μm were first decellularized by addition of DNAse and RNAse to make them non-immunogenic, in order to minimize the chances of rejection. Sodium dodecyl sulfate 0.1% is superior for decellularization, but may cause poor epithelialization.[24]

The CSE is constituted by applying fibrin glue in-between two corneal lenticules of the same donor, while maintaining the superior aspect of the lenticules upward (Fig. 12.2). These CSEs can be stored and dehydrated in glycerol for the short-term. They have been used for anterior lamellar keratoplasty in animal studies with impressive results. No corneal neovascularization, rejection or graft degradation was observed in the early postoperative period. Also, a gradual but significant reversal in transparency was noted at 3 months. After dissolution of the fibrin glue, the gap between the lenticules was also effectively replaced by the stromal keratocytes. The CSEs facilitated *in vivo* epithelial growth and adhesion with a mean delay of 16 days. This delay is proposed to be due to the lack of basement membrane over the lenticule. However, newly synthesized basement membrane and hemidesmosomes were noted after 2 months, proving that CSE can form an acceptable scaffold for epithelial growth. Long-term and human studies of this new technique are underway.

The innovations of CSE and TEKIL procedures may help in fighting the issue of donor cornea shortage in developing countries.

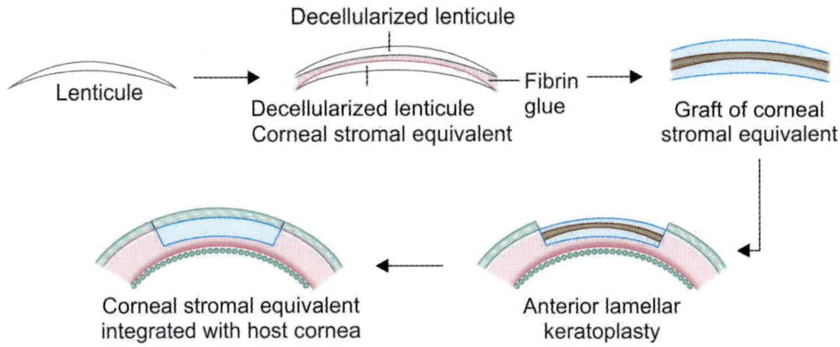

Fig. 12.2: Corneal stromal equivalents.

Epikeratophakia

Epikeratophakia is described as the application of a SMILE lenticule over the excimer treated bed of phototherapeutic keratectomy (PTK). This procedure was tried in cases of visual deterioration due to recurrence of corneal dystrophy, and an increase in the uncorrected visual acuity by greater than or equal to two lines was observed in 83% of the eyes. The short-term safety of the procedure has been established and studies are ongoing to determine its long-term effects.[22]

Management of Keratoconus Progression

This is a step ahead of the previously described FILI technique, where implantation of the lenticule is intended to treat cases of established and progressive keratoconus. The cryopreserved lenticules are retrieved based on the spherical equivalent of the patient. The lenticule is trephined in the central 3 mm to produce a donut shape. The patient's cornea is subjected to femtosecond laser to create a pocket at 100 μm depth, followed by injection of 0.25% riboflavin into the interface. After 60 seconds, the riboflavin is washed off and the donut-shaped lenticule is inserted and centered with respect to the first Purkinje image. Then UV-A radiation is applied for 3.3 minutes at 30 mW/cm^2 (total dose: 6.3 J/cm^2). The rationale to create the "donut shape" is to add tissue around the cone to cause mid-peripheral elevation, and hence relative central corneal flattening, in addition to the modification of corneal shape into a prolate or a less hyperprolate one. The 100 μm depth is optimal to cause the maximal anterior corneal effect and effective cross-linking of the cornea. This method has been observed to be effective in decreasing the overall spherical equivalent and astigmatism, but the mean keratometry (K) in cases of advanced keratoconus (K >58 D) does not change. Hence this procedure would remain more fruitful for cases of mild to moderate progressive keratoconus.[25]

Management of Post-LASIK Ectasia

Excessive tissue ablation during LASIK resulting in postsurgical ectasia can be distressing to the patient owing to the significant anisometropia induced. Such cases would typically harbor a hard to correct astigmatism too. A recent study has reported the use of a toric-myopic allogeneic lenticule implantation to manage such cases to an extent where further definitive corrective surgeries such as implantable collamer lenses may be undertaken later to achieve optimal refractive outcomes. The challenge in this type of procedure lies in the accurate alignment of the steep axis of the toric lenticule to the flat axis of the patient's cornea, after lifting the LASIK flap. It is safer to suture the flap at the end of the surgery. The study observed an overcorrection with strong myopic shift and a continuing regularization of the cornea at 3 months postoperative period. However, the ectasia was effectively treated.[26]

Collagen Cross-linking in Ultrathin Cornea—Stromal Expansion

Collagen cross-linking is a valuable option in progressive keratoconus. But its use is limited to corneas with a threshold of 400 μm stromal thickness. In cases with borderline corneal thickness, hypo-osmolar CXL, transepithelial CXL, customized debridement CXL and bandage contact lens-assisted CXL may be tried. Newer to this armamentarium is the tailored stromal expansion, which augments the patient's stromal thickness in the most physiologic way with a lenticule obtained from SMILE. The thickness of the lenticule required is decided based on the intraoperative pachymetry after epithelial debridement and can vary widely from 20 μm to 140 μm, based on the donor's refractive error. The lenticule of appropriate central thickness is positioned such that its thickest part coincides with the apex of the cone. A repeat intraoperative pachymetry is done to confirm that the augmented stromal thickness is greater than or equal to 400 μm. This is followed by CXL as per the standard Dresden protocol. After the procedure, the lenticule is removed and the stromal bed irrigated, followed by application of bandage contact lens. This procedure appears to be safe and effective.[27]

LENTICULE PRESERVATION

The use of the refractive lenticule in various tissue-additive procedures requires the development of adequate storage methods. Both short-term and long-term preservations of the refractive lenticule are being investigated.

Short-term Storage

The immediate storage of the stromal lenticule in 0.9% sodium chloride or Dulbecco's Modified Eagle's medium has been widely practiced and has not shown to have any adverse effects.[22,24] Storage in McCarey-Kaufman and corneal tissue culture medium is also well known.[18,27] The lenticule can also be temporarily stored in glycerol, especially in cases of lenticule edema, such as those post-decellularization.[24] However, for later clinical uses, special procedures for long-term preservations become mandatory.

Long-term Storage (Cryopreservation)

Dimethyl sulfoxide is used as a cryoprotectant agent for long-term cryopreservation of the refractive lenticule. The extracted SMILE lenticule is initially washed in phosphate-buffered saline (PBS) and antibiotic solution for 10 minutes, and the entire process is repeated twice. The lenticule is transferred to a cryovial containing 1 mL of 10% fetal bovine serum or tissue culture medium, along with 10% dimethyl sulfoxide. The cryovial is slowly frozen to –80°C overnight in a cryo-container and then transferred to liquid nitrogen for long-term storage. During retrieval, the vial is rapidly thawed in a water bath of 37°C, or gradually thawed by rubbing between the palms or leaving them at room temperature for 10 minutes until the medium inside liquefies.[18,28] They are then rinsed in PBS solution to relieve the lenticule of all the cryo-agents. The lenticules have been successfully preserved for up to 6 months. The viability of the cells can be confirmed by further successful tissue culture. The collagen number, structure, architecture, integrity and growth dynamics are maintained during cryopreservation, rendering the lenticules suitable for future reimplantation techniques.[28]

CONCLUSION

Innovations in medicine are a continuum. As SMILE is being widely adopted on one side for refractive correction, the endeavors in lenticule utilizations are being unwrapped on the other side. Both have been complimentary too, aiding in the management of untoward future complications using one's own tissue. Surpassing the boundaries of a simple refractive surgery, SMILE has extended its bearing onto the management of donor cornea deficits in developing nations, with an added advantage of no rejection or failure cases reported till date.[26] However, the processing and long-term preservation of the lenticule would remain a challenge. We have highlighted the current research on the diversity of the present and future applications of SMILE.

REFERENCES

1. American Society of Cataract and Refractive Surgery Meeting. (2015). Zeiss seeks FDA approval of SMILE procedure for astigmatic myopia. [online] Available from https://www.healio.com/ophthalmology/ophthalmic-business/news/online/%7B317d01ad-430e-4d38-b79d-8f2de368254e%7D/zeiss-seeks-fda-approval-of-smile-procedure-for-astigmatic-myopia. [Accessed July 2017].

2. Sekundo W, Reinstein DZ, Blum M. Improved lenticule shape for hyperopic femtosecond lenticule extraction (ReLEx® FLEx): a pilot study. Lasers Med Sci. 2016;31(4):659-64.
3. Liu YC, Ang HP, Teo EPW, et al. Wound healing profiles of hyperopic-small incision lenticule extraction (SMILE). Sci Rep. 2016;6:29802.
4. Reinstein DZ, Pradhan KR, Carp GI, et al. Small incision lenticule extraction (SMILE) for hyperopia: optical zone diameter and spherical aberration induction. J Refract Surg. 2017;33(6):370-6.
5. Ivarsen A, Hjortdal J. Correction of myopic astigmatism with small incision lenticule extraction. J Refract Surg. 2014;30(4):240-7.
6. Hansen RS, Lyhne N, Grauslund J, et al. Small-incision lenticule extraction (SMILE): outcomes of 722 eyes treated for myopia and myopic astigmatism. Graefes Arch Clin Exp Ophthalmol. 2016;254(2):399-405.
7. Jacob S, Kumar DA, Agarwal A, et al. Preliminary evidence of successful near vision enhancement with a new technique: PrEsbyopic Allogenic Refractive Lenticule (PEARL) corneal inlay using a SMILE lenticule. J Refract Surg. 2017;33(4):224-9.
8. Massoud TH, Ibrahim O, Shehata K, et al. Small incision lenticule extraction for postkeratoplasty myopia and astigmatism. J Ophthalmol. 2016;2016:e3686380.
9. Mastropasqua L, Calienno R, Lanzini M, et al. Small incision lenticule extraction after deep anterior lamellar keratoplasty. J Refract Surg. 2015;31(9):634-7.
10. Zhang S, Xu H, Zheng K, et al. The observation during small incision lenticule extraction for myopia with corneal opacity. BMC Ophthalmol. 2017;17:80.
11. Ganesh S, Brar S. Clinical outcomes of small incision lenticule extraction with accelerated cross-linking (ReLEx SMILE Xtra) in patients with thin corneas and borderline topography. J Ophthalmol. 2015;2015:263412.
12. Ng AL, Chan TC, Cheng GP, et al. Comparison of the early clinical outcomes between combined small-incision lenticule extraction and collagen cross-linking versus SMILE for myopia. J Ophthalmol. 2016;2016:e2672980.
13. Graue-Hernandez EO, Pagano GL, Garcia-De la Rosa G, et al. Combined small-incision lenticule extraction and intrastromal corneal collagen crosslinking to treat mild keratoconus: long-term follow-up. J Cataract Refract Surg. 2015;41(11):2524-32.
14. Catalan-Lopez S, Portas-Ferradas AM, Cadarso-Suarez L, et al. Small incision lenticule extraction (SMILE) as retreatment for a thick LASIK flap. J Refract Surg. 2016;32(10):718-20.
15. European Society of Cataract and Refractive Surgeons. (2016). Retreatment strategies following small incision lenticule extraction (SMILE): in vivo tissue response and clinical results. [online] Available from http://www.escrs.org/Copenhagen2016/programme/poster-village-details.asp?id=26674&day=0. [Accessed July 2017].
16. Donate D, Thaëron R. Preliminary evidence of successful enhancement after a primary SMILE procedure with the sub-cap-lenticule-extraction technique. J Refract Surg. 2015;31(10):708-10.
17. European Society of Cataract and Refractive Surgeons. (2016). Capless SMILE: an intrastromal option for retreatment after ReLEx® SMILE. [online] Available from http://www.escrs.org/Copenhagen2016/programme/free-papers-details.asp?id=27010&day=0. [Accessed July 2017].
18. Ganesh S, Brar S, Rao PA. Cryopreservation of extracted corneal lenticules after small incision lenticule extraction for potential use in human subjects. Cornea. 2014;33(12):1355-62.

19. Sun L, Yao P, Li M, et al. The safety and predictability of implanting autologous lenticule obtained by SMILE for hyperopia. J Refract Surg. 2015;31(6):374-9.
20. Angunawela RI, Riau AK, Chaurasia SS, et al. Refractive lenticule re-implantation after myopic ReLEx: a feasibility study of stromal restoration after refractive surgery in a rabbit model. Invest Ophthalmol Vis Sci. 2012;53(8):4975-85.
21. Pradhan KR, Reinstein DZ, Carp GI, et al. Femtosecond laser-assisted keyhole endokeratophakia: correction of hyperopia by implantation of an allogeneic lenticule obtained by SMILE from a myopic donor. J Refract Surg. 2013;29(11):777-82.
22. Jiang Y, Li Y, Liu X-W, et al. A novel tectonic keratoplasty with femtosecond laser intrastromal lenticule for corneal ulcer and perforation. Chin Med J (Engl). 2016;129(15):1817-21.
23. Xue C, Xia Y, Chen Y, et al. Treatment of large corneal perforations with acellular multilayer of corneal stromal lenticules harvested from femtosecond laser lenticule extraction. Zhonghua Yan Ke Za Zhi. 2015;51(9):655-9.
24. Yin H, Qiu P, Wu F, et al. Construction of a corneal stromal equivalent with SMILE-derived lenticules and fibrin glue. Sci Rep. 2016;6:33848.
25. Ganesh S, Brar S. Femtosecond intrastromal lenticular implantation combined with accelerated collagen cross-linking for the treatment of keratoconus—initial clinical result in 6 eyes. Cornea. 2015;34(10):1331-9.
26. Lazaridis A, Messerschmidt-Roth A, Sekundo W, et al. Refractive lenticule implantation for correction of ametropia: case reports and literature review. Klin Monatsbl Augenheilkd. 2017;234(1):77-89.
27. Sachdev MS, Gupta D, Sachdev G, et al. Tailored stromal expansion with a refractive lenticule for crosslinking the ultrathin cornea. J Cataract Refract Surg. 2015;41(5):918-23.
28. Mohamed-Noriega K, Toh KP, Poh R, et al. Cornea lenticule viability and structural integrity after refractive lenticule extraction (ReLEx) and cryopreservation. Mol Vis. 2011;17:3437-49.

Index

Page numbers followed by *f* refer to figure, *fc* refer to flow chart, *t* refer to table.

A

Aberration, higher-order 12, 17, 159
Ablation zone diameter 149
Accurate centration 126
Acne vulgaris, treatment of 11
Allograft 167
Ambrósio relational thickness 15
Anterior segment optical coherence tomography 89, 100, 105*f*, 107*f*, 120, 121, 139, 140
ASOCT *See* Anterior segment optical coherence tomography
Astigmatic keratotomy 5
Astigmatism 16
Autograft 167
Automated lamellar keratoplasty 2

B

Balanced salt solution 49
Barraquer-Krumeich-Swinger 2
  nonfreeze technique 3
BCVA See Best corrected visual acuity
Belin-Ambrósio enhanced ectasia display 15
Best corrected visual acuity 10, 12, 115, 164
Black spots 94, 95, 100
  prevention 95
Bowman's layer 119

C

Cap cut 54
Cap microstriae 114, 118
  management 119
  pathophysiology 119
Cap parameters 40, 54*f*
Cap side-cut 55
Cap-lenticular adhesion
  case of 107*f*
  sinskey hook 101*f*
Carl Zeiss contact lens 88
Centration 73
Chung's swing technique 59
Cleavage planes, dissection of 73
Collagen cross-linking 161, 170
Contact glass interface, treatment pack with 35*f*
Contact lens 50*f*, 94*f*
  related factors 95
Contrast sensitivity 13, 78, 83
Corneal
  biomechanical strength 78, 85
  biomechanics 153, 154
  clarity 78, 83
  ectasia 130
  hysteresis 27, 78, 85, 153
  innervation 155
  keratocyte density 24
  light reflex, coaxially sighted 51
  nerve fiber
    anatomy of 23
    layer changes 24
  pachymetry 15, 153
  refractive surgery 3
    evolution of 2*fc*
  resistance factor 27, 78, 85, 153
  sensations 29, 78, 84
  stromal equivalent 168, 169*f*
  sub-basal nerve fibers 25*f*
  topography 15, 152
    regular 152
  vertex centration 129
  visualization Scheimpflug technology 22, 27
  wound healing 21
    cascade 21
    postoperative 21
Corrected distance visual acuity 79
Corvis ST See Corneal visualization Scheimpflug technology
Cryopreservation 171
Curvilinear lenticulerrhexis, continuous 58, 103

D

Dense opaque bubble layer 96*f*
Diabetes mellitus 10
Diffuse lamellar keratitis 115, 131
  pathophysiology 131
Docking 52*f*, 73
  related factors 95
Dry eye 114, 118, 154
  management 118
  pathophysiology 118
  prevention 118
  syndrome 14

E

Ectasia 115, 130
  management 131
  pathophysiology 130
  risk score system 15
Endokeratophakia 167
Epidermal growth factor 21
Epikeratophakia 169
Epithelial defect 110
  during surgery 120
  extent of 105*f*
  management 110
Epithelial ingrowth 114, 119
  diagnosis of 121
  pathophysiology 119
Eyes, number of 79

F

Femtosecond laser
  application 49, 53, 69*f*, 96*f*
  delivery 52*f*, 67*f*, 145*f*, 162
  in corneal refractive surgery 4
  intrastromal lenticular
    implantation 167
    tectonic keratoplasty with 167
  settings and treatment parameters 53*f*
  technology 6, 148
    evolution of 1
Femtosecond laser-assisted in situ keratomileusis 9, 65, 148, 154
Femtosecond lenticule extraction 10, 28, 32, 68, 68*f*, 99, 103, 146
Fixation ring 62*f*
FLEx See Femtosecond lenticule extraction
FS-LASIK See Femtosecond laser-assisted in situ keratomileusis
Fundus examination 14

G

Glaucoma 1

H

Herpes infection 11
Hyperopia 16, 161
  surgical correction of 161
  treatment of 167
Hyperopic lenticule 162, 163*f*
Hyperopic refractive correction 18
Hyperopic SMILE lenticule 162*t*

I

Immune-deficient states 10
In situ keratomileusis 3
Infectious keratitis 132
  management 133
Inflammatory mediators 28
Infrared illumination 37
Interface debris 132
Interface haze 113, 114
  management 117
  pathophysiology 113
  prevention 117
Intraocular pressure 5, 26, 149, 150
  preoperative 15
Intraoperative manipulations, increased 124
Intraoperative signs 103
Intraoperative suction loss 90*t*, 138
  management of 92*fc*
Intrastromal lenticule 67*f*, 68*f*
Irregular topography 114, 123
  management 124

K

Keratitis, infective 115
Keratoconus 130
  progression, management of 169
Keratoplasty 5
Kyphosis 12

L

Lamellar dissectors 60*f*
LASER See Light amplification by stimulated emission of radiation
Laser
  arm 36
  in ophthalmology 1
  keratome 35*f*

parameters for small incision lenticule extraction 42*t*
settings 99, 124
selection of 41
spots depicting spot distance 43*f*
Laser-assisted
in situ keratomileusis 4, 16, 22, 92, 113, 115, 141, 142, 149*t*, 154*t*, 159*f*
postoperative 155*f*
subepithelial keratomileusis 2
Laser-induced optical breakdown 32, 95
LASIK See Laser-assisted in situ keratomileusis
Lenticule
characteristics 99, 100, 162
creation sequence and time 162
cut 54
diameter 39
dissection 99, 102
difficult 139
management of difficult 100*fc*
pathophysiology of difficult 100*fc*
dissection and extraction 36, 49, 55
modified techniques for 55
pathophysiology of difficult 98*f*
edge identification 74*f*
extraction
anatomical effects of 104*f*
difficult 89, 97
management, difficult 100
microforceps for 61*f*
pathophysiology, difficult 98
physiological effects of difficult 104*f*
sub-cap 141, 145, 166
minimum thickness of 40
parameters 38, 39*f*, 40
preservation 170
side-cut 54
stripper 62*f*
thickness 131
Light amplification by stimulated emission of radiation 1
Lims corneoscleral forceps 62, 63*f*
LIOB See Laser-induced optical breakdown
Low-suction system 90

M

Manifest refraction spherical equivalent 78, 82, 149, 161
MASER See Microwave amplification by stimulated emission of radiation
Mitomycin C 115
MRSE See Manifest refraction spherical equivalent
Myopia 161
and myopic astigmatism 79*t*-82*t*
high 79, 81, 82, 130
low 79, 81, 82
with astigmatism 79, 81
with corneal opacity 164
Myopic 162*t*
astigmatism 163
lenticule 162

N

Neodymium-doped yttrium lithium fluoride 4
Nerve fiber layer, preoperative sub-basal 156*f*
Nerve growth factor 28

O

Ocular
adnexal examination 13
allergic disease 11
ectatic diseases 11
examination 13
comprehensive 12
motility assessment 13
response analyzer 22, 27, 78, 85, 154
surface
disease index 22, 29, 78, 85
disease, mild 16
disorders 17
examination 14
stability 29, 155
surface-related
factors 95
problems 154
Opaque bubble layer 89, 95, 99, 108, 115, 124
management 97
Optical aberrations 78, 83, 115, 125
management 125
Optical zone 38
diameter 149
OSDI See Ocular surface disease index

P

Palpebral fissures, small 17
Paracentral cap tear 106*f*

Patient supporting system 36
PEARL See Presbyopic allogenic refractive lenticule
Pellucid marginal degeneration 11
Peripheral small abrasions 110
Photorefractive keratectomy 2, 3, 26, 13, 89, 115, 140, 141, 142, 154, 155, 164
Phototherapeutic keratectomy 2
Postkeratoplasty refractive correction 164
Post-LASIK ectasia, management of 170
Post-SMILE
  enhancement 145*f*
    and retreatment 137
  retreatment, decision-making in 140*fc*
Potential visual complaints of blurred vision 124*f*
Presbyopia 163
Presbyopic allogenic refractive lenticule 163
PRK See Photorefractive keratectomy
Pseudo-small incision lenticule extraction 69, 69*f*
Pulse energy
  decreased 44
  increased 44
  on small incision lenticule extraction 44*t*
Pupillary examination 14

R

Refraction 13
Refractive applications of SMILE, expanding 161
Refractive error 11, 100, 151
  higher 16
  magnitude of 72, 138
Refractive lenticule 67*f*
  extraction 77
    flap-based 66
    flapless 148
    wet-lab training for 67*f*
  of SMILE, applications of 166
Refractive outcomes 77, 154, 156
Refractive surgery 1, 16*t*
Reimplantation techniques 171
Residual stromal bed thickness 41, 115, 139, 140, 149
  low 130
Retained lenticule 89, 108, 109
  management 109
  prevention 108
Retinal tears 11
Rigid gas permeables 11
RSBT See Residual stromal bed thickness

S

Schirmer's test 118
Scoliosis 12
Seibel spatula 68f
Shimmer sign 55, 58
Sinskey hook-assisted lenticule extraction 101*f*
Slit illumination 37
Slit-lamp examination 14
Small incision lenticule extraction 9, 9*t*, 12, 16, 16*t*, 21, 22*t*, 25*f*, 26*f*, 32, 38*t*, 39*f*, 46, 47*t*, 49*t*, 52*f*, 56*f*, 58*t*, 65, 66, 66*t*, 70, 71*t*, 77, 88, 89*t*, 99, 105, 113, 114*t*, 137, 142*f*, 148, 149*t*, 154*t*, 156*f*, 161
  biomechanical
    changes after 26
    properties after 27
  cap parameters for 39*f*
  case of 96*f*
  differs from lasik 148
  efficacy of 79*t*
  epithelial 61
  for re-treatment after refractive surgery 166
  forceps 61
  functional changes after 29
  healing cascade after 23*fc*
  in hyperopia 83
  in thick-flap lasik 166
  lamellar dissectors 59
  lenticule 107*f*
    strippers 62
  performing 45*t*
  physiological outcomes of 78*t*
  postoperative 155*f*
    complications in 113
  predictability of 81*t*
  pros and cons of 159*f*
  refractive outcomes of 78*t*
  repeat 166
  retreatment after 141*t*
  safety of 80*t*
  stability of 82*t*
  starburst in left eye after 124*f*
  stepwise learning curve of 66*f*
  surgical instruments during 60*f*
  surgical technique of 46
  treatment parameters for 40*t*

SMILE See Small incision lenticule extraction
Spherical aberrations 14
Spherical powers 149
Stromal expansion 170
Stromal keratocyte density, anterior 26*f*
Stromal lenticule, storage of 170
Stromal nerve plexus, anterior 24
Suction loss 88, 138
  management 92
  pathophysiology 88
  prevention 91
Surgical instruments 59
Surgical procedure 149

T

TBUT See Tear film breakup time
Tear
  meniscus 52*f*
  side-cut 89, 106*f*
Tear film
  breakup time 12, 22, 78
  changes 78
  stability 84
Technolas perfect vision 5
Thin-flap lasik 142
Tonometry 15
Topical anesthesia 95
Total lenticule thickness 40
Traumatic dislocation of flaps 17

U

UDVA See Uncorrected distance visual acuity
Ultrathin cornea 170
Uncorrected distance visual acuity 78
Uncorrected visual acuity 10, 12
Universal wire speculum 62, 63*f*
Uveitis 11

V

Vacuum system 36
Visual
  acuity 13, 77, 78, 157
    uncorrected distance 79, 165
  function analysis 124*f*
  quality 78, 82, 157
  recovery 154, 156
    time 78, 82
VisuMax femtosecond laser system 32, 33*f*, 40*t*
  components of 34*t*
  functional components of 34*f*
  technical specifications of 45*t*
VisuMax femtosecond laser-assisted small incision 161
VisuMax laser 5, 145*f*
  circle pattern of 143, 144*f*
VisuMax system 164

W

Weighing pros and cons 158
Wet-lab training 67
White-ring sign 58, 103

Y

Y-shaped instrument 62